Ophthalmic Pocket Companion

D1292105

Ophthalmic Pocket Companion

Fifth Edition

Dean Dornic, O.D., M.D.
Private Practice, Raleigh, North Carolina

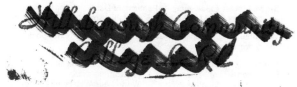

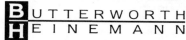

BUTTERWORTH
HEINEMANN

Boston   Oxford   Johannesburg   Melbourne   New Delhi   Singapore

Library of Congress Cataloging-in-Publication Data
Dornic, Dean.
     Ophthalmic pocket companion / Dean Dornic. -- 5th ed.
          p.   cm.
     Includes bibliographical references and index.
     ISBN 0-7506-7120-3
     1. Ophthalmology--Handbooks, manuals, etc.   I. Title
     [DNLM: 1. Eye Diseases handbooks.   2. Pharmaceutical Preparations
handbooks.   3. Eye--drug effects handbooks.   WW 39 D714o 1999]
     RE48.9.D67   1999
     617.7--dc21
     DNLM/DLC
     for Library of Congress   98-37681
                                                                                                              CIP

British Library Cataloguing-in-Publication Data
A catalogue record for this book is available from the British Library.

The publisher offers special discounts on bulk orders of this book.
For information, please write:

Manager of Special Sales   For information on all B-H
Butterworth–Heinemann   publications available, contact our
225 Wildwood Avenue   World Wide Web home page at:
Woburn, MA 01801–2041   http://www.bh.com
Tel: 781-904-2500
Fax: 781-904-2620

10 9 8 7 6 5 4 3 2 1

Printed in the United States of America

To my wife Pamela and my children
Matthew, Jevin, and Elyssa

Contents

Preface

I am continually amazed at how rapidly things change in the eye care field. The previous edition of the *Ophthalmic Pocket Companion* was published only 3 years ago, yet the number of revisions necessary for this new fifth edition is incredible. In addition to revising every chapter, I have included many new topics. The discussions of orbital disease and pediatrics have especially been strengthened. I have deleted the contact lens section under the assumption that most practitioners have other resources for this information, which becomes dated very quickly. I have also added sections on ocular syndromes, typical laser settings, and abbreviations. Please personalize this book with your own notes, and, as always, I encourage you to share comments about the book with me.

DEAN DORNIC

Differential Diagnosis of Ocular Signs and Symptoms

Anisocoria (Unequal Pupils) (see Chap. 10)

Band Keratopathy

Hypercalcemia
Chronic uveitis
Phthisis bulbi
Interstitial keratitis
Gout
Corneal dystrophies
Renal failure
Long-standing glaucoma
Exposure to irritants (long-standing)
Viscoat use

Blepharospasm (Bilateral Uncontrollable Blinking) (see also Chap. 4)

Psychogenic
Pain from foreign body, keratitis, etc.
Idiopathic (essential blepharospasm)
Tourette's syndrome
Parkinson's disease
Encephalitis
Drugs

Burning

Blepharitis
Dry eye/surface abnormality
Keratoconjunctivitis
Episcleritis

Cataract (Posterior Subcapsular)

Steroid use
Chronic iritis
Retinitis pigmentosa
Diabetes mellitus
Ocular trauma
Idiopathic
Myotonic dystrophy
Fabry's disease
Ionizing radiation
Systemic syndromes (e.g., Pierre Robin syndrome)

Conjunctivitis (Acute)

Bacterial
Viral
Allergic/toxic
Foreign body/trauma
Contact lens/giant papillary conjunctivitis

Conjunctivitis (Chronic)

Medicamentosa
Dry eye/surface abnormality
Chlamydia
Thyroid eye disease
Blepharoconjunctivitis
Dacryocystitis
Spring allergies

Ocular pemphigoid
Rosacea
Phlyctenulosis
Angular blepharoconjunctivitis
Parinaud's conjunctivitis

Corneal Crystals

Crystalline dystrophy of Schnyder
Bietti marginal crystalline dystrophy
Gout
Uremia
Hyperparathyroidism
Cholesterol (with vascularization) after trauma or infection
Cystinosis
Waldenström's disease
Multiple myeloma
Postkeratoplasty
Drugs (e.g., chloroquine, thioridazine hydrochloride [Mellaril])

Corneal Edema

Contact lens overwear
Fuchs' dystrophy
Aphakic bullous keratopathy
Trauma
Early postoperative
Glaucoma
Hydrops (keratoconus)
Herpes simplex (disciform)
Herpes zoster (disciform)
Acanthamoeba
Iritis
Iridocorneal endothelial syndrome

Corneal Opacity (Whorl-Like)

Vortex dystrophy
Amiodarone
Fabry's disease
Chloroquine
Phenothiazines
Indomethacin

Corneal Punctate Lesions (Keratopathy)

Dry eyes (keratitis sicca)
Adenovirus
Contact lens related
Medicamentosa
Blepharitis
Bacterial conjunctivitis
Exposure
Chlamydia
Herpes simplex
Molluscum contagiosum
Warts
Benign mucous membrane pemphigoid
Erythema multiforme
Radiation injury
Superior limbic keratoconjunctivitis
Ocular rosacea
Reiter's disease
Trichiasis (inturned lashes)
Ectropion
Entropion
Drugs

Corneal (Stromal) Ring Infiltrate

Acanthamoeba keratitis
Anesthetic abuse keratopathy

Herpes simplex keratitis
Bacillus cereus keratitis
Capnocytophagia keratitis
Gram-negative endotoxin reaction

Cotton-Wool Spots

Diabetes
Hypertension
Systemic lupus erythematosus
Retinal vascular occlusion
Human immunodeficiency virus (HIV)
Carotid artery disease
Purtscher's retinopathy (after crush injury to chest or long bones)
Anemia
Leukemia
Lymphoma

Dacryoadenitis (Inflammation of the Lacrimal Gland)

Measles
Mumps
Influenza
Infectious mononucleosis
Typhoid fever
Gonorrhea
Scarlet fever
Secondary to conjunctivitis, uveitis, etc.
Sarcoidosis
Tuberculosis
Brucellosis
Leukemia
Lymphoma
Pseudotumor
Syphilis
Neoplasm (e.g., adenoma)

Distorted Vision (Metamorphopsia)

Macular degeneration
Central serous maculopathy
Retinal pigment epithelium detachment
Retinal detachment
Macular hemorrhage/edema
Corneal irregularity
Retinal dystrophy
Cataract (generally not true metamorphopsia)
Refractive error (generally not true metamorphopsia)

Double Vision (see Chap. 10)

Dry Eyes (see Chap. 4)

Ectopia Lentis (see Subluxated Lens)

Emboli (Retinal)

Platelet and fibrin
Hollenhorst plaque (cholesterol)
Calcium (cardiac)
Talc (in intravenous drug abuse)
Lipid (Purtscher's retinopathy; seen after crush injuries to chest or
    long bones)
Tumor (e.g., cardiac myxoma)
Foreign body

Epiphora (see Tearing)

Episcleral Injection (Dilated Vessels)

Carotid cavernous fistula
Underlying uveal melanoma
Ophthalmic vein or cavernous sinus thrombosis
Polycythemia vera
Leukemia
Thyroid eye disease

Exophthalmos

Thyroid eye disease
Pseudotumor
Orbital tumor/mass
Carotid cavernous fistula
Severe myopia
Pseudoexophthalmos (enophthalmos or ptosis in fellow eye, facial
   asymmetry)

Extraocular Muscle Enlargement

Thyroid eye disease
Pseudotumor
Metastatic carcinoma
Arteriovenous fistula
Collagen vascular disease
Cysticercosis
Trichinosis
Acromegaly

Eyelash Loss (Madarosis)

Staphylococcal blepharitis
Skin disorders (e.g., psoriasis, dermatophytosis, neurodermatitis)
Sebaceous gland carcinoma
Drugs
Endocrine disease (e.g., hypothyroidism)
Vogt-Koyanagi-Harada syndrome
Radiation
Severe systemic disease (e.g., tuberculosis, leprosy, syphilis)
Idiopathic

Facial Palsy

Bell's palsy (idiopathic)
Herpes zoster

Basal skull fracture
Congenital (e.g., trauma, Möbius' syndrome)
Otitis media
Central/nuclear (e.g., stroke, tumor)
Neoplasm (e.g., schwannoma, parotid tumor)
Sarcoidosis
Diabetes mellitus
Lyme disease
Guillain-Barré syndrome
Klippel-Feil syndrome

Filamentary Keratitis

Dry eyes (keratitis sicca)
Recurrent erosion
Neurotrophic keratitis
Medicamentosa

Flashing Lights

Retinal traction (e.g., tear, posterior vitreous detachment)
Migraine (usually minutes rather than seconds)
Rapid eye movements (in dark)
Intracranial mass or lesion

Foreign Body Sensation

Foreign body (under lid)
Dry eye
Blepharitis
Keratitis
Conjunctivitis
Exposure
Pinguecula/pterygium
Recurrent corneal erosion
Superficial punctate keratitis of Thygeson

Superior limbic keratoconjunctivitis
Episcleritis
Contact lens or solution problem

Giant Papillary Conjunctivitis

Contact lens related
Foreign body related (e.g., sutures, under lid)
Ocular prosthesis
Vernal conjunctivitis
Atopic keratoconjunctivitis

Hallucinations (Visual)

Migraine
Posterior vitreous detachment (illusion)
Retinal detachment (illusion)
Vitreal floaters/opacities (illusion)
Schizophrenia
Other psychiatric disorders
Drugs
Hypnagogic hallucinations

Halos Around Lights

Acute angle closure glaucoma
Other causes of high intraocular pressure
Refractive error
Cataract
Corneal edema/problem

Headache

Tension
Migraine
Cluster

Giant cell arteritis
Acute glaucoma
Eye strain/refractive error
Hypertension
Increased intracranial pressure
Meningitis
Sinus disease
Subarachnoid hemorrhage
Postherpetic neuralgia
Temporomandibular joint syndrome
Dental disorders
Trigeminal neuralgia
Anterior uveitis
Psychogenic

Heterochromia Iridis (Color Differs Between Eyes)

Congenital Horner's syndrome
Fuchs' heterochromic iridocyclitis
Intraocular foreign body
Nevus
Melanoma
Chronic uveitis
Metastatic carcinoma
Waardenburg's syndrome
Retinoblastoma
Iridocorneal endothelial syndrome
Neurofibromas

Hyphema (Blood in Anterior Chamber)

Trauma
Intraocular surgery
Iris neovascularization
Herpes simplex or zoster iritis
Blood dyscrasias

Hemophilia
Intraocular tumor
Juvenile xanthogranuloma

Iris Lesions

Nevus
Melanoma
Iris cyst
Granuloma
Neurofibroma
Metastatic carcinoma
Foreign body

Iris Neovascularization

Diabetes mellitus
Central retinal vein occlusion
Branch retinal vein occlusion
Carotid artery disease
Melanoma
Metastatic carcinoma
Anterior chamber implants
Fungal endophthalmitis
Chronic uveitis
Postretinal detachment surgery
Takayasu's syndrome (aortic arch syndrome)
Coats' disease
Eales' disease
Chronic open angle glaucoma
Retinal detachment
Retinoblastoma
Sickle cell retinopathy
Giant cell arteritis
Postvitrectomy
Sympathetic ophthalmia

Leukokoria (White Pupil)

Cataract
Retinoblastoma
Coats' disease
Coloboma of choroid
Medullated nerve fibers
Endophthalmitis
Ocular toxocariasis
Persistent hyperplastic primary vitreous
Organized vitreous hemorrhage
Retinopathy of prematurity
Toxoplasmosis
Retinal dysplasia
Exudative retinitis
Congenital retinal detachment
Juvenile retinoschisis
Retinal astrocytoma

Lid Myokymia

Fatigue
Caffeine (excess or withdrawal)
Debilitating diseases
Anemia
Excessive alcohol or smoking
Trigeminal neuralgia
Irritative anterior segment disorder
Multiple sclerosis
Myasthenia gravis

Lid Retraction

Hyperthyroidism
Associated ptosis of fellow eye

Sylvian aqueduct syndrome
Aberrent regeneration of third nerve
Midbrain lesion
Duane's retraction syndrome
Brown's vertical retraction syndrome
Hydrocephalus
Meningitis
Drugs
Multiple sclerosis
Parkinson's disease
Syphilis
Malingering/hysteria
Lid scarring
Craniostenosis
Marcus Gunn's jaw-winking syndrome

Lid Swelling (Inflammatory)

Hordeolum, chalazion
Urticaria from drugs
Associated with bacterial or viral conjunctivitis
Contact (allergic) dermatitis
Dacryoadenitis
Insect bites
Preseptal or orbital cellulitis

Lid Swelling (Noninflammatory)

Angioneurotic edema from drugs (e.g., aspirin, penicillin)
Chalazion
Systemic edema (e.g., cardiac or renal disease)
Dermatochalasis (loose eyelid skin)
Prolapse of orbital fat
Tumor

Lid Twitching

Myokymia (see Lid Myokymia)
Ocular irritation (e.g., keratitis)
Benign essential blepharospasm
Blepharospasm associated with tardive dyskinesia (drug induced)
Blepharospasm associated with central nervous system abnormalities
  (e.g., brain stem lesion)
Hemifacial spasm
Psychogenic

Light Sensitivity

Ocular inflammation (e.g., keratitis, uveitis)
Aniridia
Lightly pigmented eye (including albinism)
Migraine
Meningitis
Achromatopsia (total color blindness)
Drugs (e.g., digitoxin, amiodarone)
Psychogenic

Madarosis

Psoriasis
Neurodermatitis
Alopecia areata
Lupus erythematosus
Congenital
Drugs
Thyroid disease
Blepharitis
Sebaceous gland carcinoma
Radiation
Vogt-Koyanagi-Harada syndrome
Trauma
Syphilis

Leprosy
Sickle cell anemia

Membranous Conjunctivitis

Streptococcus
Pneumococcus
Corynebacterium diphtheriae
Adenovirus
Ligneous conjunctivitis

Metamorphopsia (see Distorted Vision)

Night Blindness

Refractive error
Miotic pupils
Cataracts
Retinitis pigmentosa
Vitamin A deficiency
Glaucoma
Drugs
Gyrate atrophy
Choroideremia
Congenital stationary night blindness

Nystagmus

Congenital idiopathic
Associated with reduced vision (e.g., aniridia, Leber's congenital
    amaurosis, achromotopsia)
Toxic/metabolic (e.g., Wernicke's encephalopathy, lithium, barbitu-
    rates)
Cerebral vascular accident
Multiple sclerosis
Tumor (usually posterior fossa)
Trauma

Vestibular lesion
Physiologic (end gaze, optokinetic)

Optic Nerve Atrophy

Glaucoma
Following optic neuritis
Following ischemic optic neuropathy
Central retinal artery occlusion
Trauma
Tobacco or alcohol (nutritional) amblyopia
Drugs (e.g., ethambutol)
Hereditary (e.g., Leber's hereditary optic neuropathy, dominant
    optic atrophy)
Compressive lesions (e.g., retrobulbar mass)
Syphilis

Optociliary Shunt Vessels

Meningioma
Other tumors
Chronic open-angle glaucoma
Chronic papilledema
After central retinal vein occlusion

Painful Eye (No Obvious Inflammation)

Retrobulbar neuritis
High intraocular pressure
Sinus disease
Refractive error
Heterophoria/heterotropia
Headache/referred pain

Pannus

Contact lenses (hypoxia or exposure)
Chlamydia

Superior limbic keratoconjunctivitis
Staphylococcal hypersensitivity
Vernal conjunctivitis
Herpes simplex keratitis
Ocular rosacea

Peripheral Retinal Neovascularization

Sickling hemoglobinopathies
Diabetes mellitus
Branch retinal vein occlusion
Retinopathy of prematurity
Eales' disease
Hyperviscosity syndromes
Aortic arch syndrome
Sarcoidosis
Uveitis
Dominant exudative vitreoretinopathy
Retinal embolization
Carotid cavernous fistula
Systemic lupus erythematosus
Retinal vasculitis
Norrie's disease
Incontinentia pigmenti

Photophobia (Light Sensitivity)

Corneal abrasion
Keratitis
Iritis
Albinism
Lightly pigmented eye
Aniridia
Migraine
Meningitis
Subarachnoid hemorrhage
Retrobulbar optic neuritis

Trigeminal neuralgia
Drugs

Poliosis (Whitening of Lashes and Hair)

Aging
Albinism
Vitiligo
Vogt-Koyanagi-Harada syndrome
Alopecia areata
Drugs
Radiation
Waardenburg's syndrome
Severe dermatitis
Idiopathic

Ptosis

Congenital
Trauma
Horner's syndrome
Oculomotor nerve palsy
Myasthenia gravis
Senility
Drugs (e.g., phenobarbital, prednisone)
Prolonged topical steroid use
Protective ptosis (after injury)
Tumor
Giant papillary conjunctivitis, vernal conjunctivitis, and other conditions of lid
Pseudoptosis (as from enophthalmos, dermatochalasis, etc.)

Punctate Keratitis

Dry eye
Exposure

Toxic (e.g., medicamentosa)
Blepharitis
Adenovirus
Herpes simplex
Chlamydia
Bacterial keratoconjunctivitis
Superior limbic keratoconjunctivitis
Superficial punctate keratitis of Thygeson
Vernal conjunctivitis
Molluscum contagiosum
Acne rosacea
Benign mucous membrane pemphigoid
Corneal dystrophies

Refractive Error Changes

Diabetes mellitus
Nuclear cataract (myopic shift most common)
Ciliary spasm
Medications (e.g., betamethasone, methacholine)
Dislocated lens
Retinal detachment/retinal pigment epithelium detachment (hyperopic shift)
Central serous chorioretinopathy (hyperopic shift)
Corneal scars
Contact lens induced
Keratoconus

Retinal Hemorrhages

Diabetes mellitus
Systemic hypertension
Retinal vein occlusion
Blood dyscrasias (e.g., cryoglobulinemia, thrombocytopenia, macroglobulinemia, polycythemia vera)

Trauma
Anemias (including those secondary to drugs)
Leukemia
Inflammatory conditions (e.g., subacute bacterial endocarditis)
Septic retinitis
Sickle cell anemia
Eales' disease
Macular degeneration (wet)
Optic nerve drusen
Preeclampsia
Arteriosclerosis
Subarachnoid hemorrhage
Venous stasis (as in carotid insufficiency)
Collagen vascular disease (e.g., lupus, scleroderma)
Infectious disease (e.g., cytomegalovirus, typhus, malaria)
Retinal macroaneurysm

Retinal Neovascularization

Diabetes
After central or branch vein occlusion
Eales' disease
Sickle cell retinopathy
Beta thalassemia
Retinopathy of prematurity
Retinal embolization (e.g., talc)
Familial exudative vitreoretinopathy
Hyperviscosity syndromes (e.g., chronic myelogenous leukemia)
Ocular ischemic syndromes (aortic arch/carotid artery disease)
Carotid cavernous fistula
Toxemia of pregnancy
Encircling scleral buckle
Multiple sclerosis

Retinal Pigment Clumping (Bone Spicules)

Retinitis pigmentosa
Chorioretinitis (e.g., syphilis)
Trauma
Rubella
Other viral infections
Senile pigmentary changes
After retinal detachment
Vitamin A deficiency
Phenothiazines
Old vascular occlusion
Retinopathy of prematurity
Cystinosis

Retinal Vasculitis

Systemic lupus erythematosus
Multiple sclerosis
Polyarteritis nodosa
Behçet's disease
Temporal arteritis
Wegener's syndrome (granulomatosis)
Sarcoidosis
Herpes zoster
Syphilis
Toxoplasmosis
Eales' disease
Cytomegalovirus retinitis
Acute retinal necrosis
Progressive outer retinal necrosis (minimal vasculitis)

Retinal Vein Occlusions (see Chap. 14)

Roth's Spots (White, Centered Hemorrhages)

Leukemia

Endocarditis
Diabetes
Anemia
Sickle cell disease
Systemic lupus erythematosus

Subluxated (Dislocated) Lens

Marfan's syndrome
Trauma
Homocystinuria
Syphilis
Ehlers-Danlos syndrome
Weill-Marchesani syndrome
Rieger's syndrome
Treacher-Collins syndrome
Apert's syndrome
Capsular exfoliation syndrome
Marchesani's syndrome
Hyperlysinemia
Simple hereditary

Subretinal Neovascular Membrane

Macular degeneration
Histoplasmosis
Best's macular degeneration
Trauma (after choroidal rupture)
Myopia
Neoplasm
Angioid streaks
Optic nerve drusen
Photocoagulation
Retinitis pigmentosa
Doyne's honeycombed dystrophy

Tearing (Epiphora)

Response to pain (e.g., foreign body, keratitis, abrasion, iritis)
Reflex (as in dry eye)
Nasolacrimal duct or punctal occlusion
Poor apposition of lid to globe (e.g., senile, injury, scarring, ectropion)

Uveitis (see Chap. 6)

Vision Loss (Gradual)

Refractive error
Cataract
Age-related macular degeneration
Glaucoma
Diabetic retinopathy
Corneal dystrophy/keratoconus
Tumor along visual pathway
Functional

Vision Loss (Sudden)

Central retinal artery occlusion
Retinal vein occlusion
Vitreous hemorrhage
Retinal detachment
Optic neuritis
Ischemic optic neuropathy
Acute glaucoma
Uveitis/choroiditis
Cerebral vascular accident (bilateral)
Functional

Vision Loss (Transient)

Amaurosis fugax (monocular [minutes])
Vertebrobasilar artery insufficiency (binocular [minutes])

Papilledema (seconds)
Migraine (minutes)
Systemic hypotension (often seen with change in posture)
Heart failure
Anemia
Impending retinal vascular occlusion
Giant cell arteritis
Uhtoff's syndrome (in demyelinating disease)
Glaucoma
Optic nerve drusen

NOTES

2

Ocular Trauma

Ocular trauma can occur in isolation or in association with injury to multiple organ systems. The nature of the injury dictates the type of ancillary testing required. In any case, a thorough eye examination with particular attention to function and structures vulnerable to the type of trauma is mandatory. Some of the more common eye injuries are discussed in this chapter.

ECCHYMOSIS (BLACK EYE)

No treatment is necessary. Resolves in approximately 2 weeks. Look for more significant sequelae to injury. May suggest the following to hasten recovery:

- Cold compresses for the first 24 hours to limit bruising and reduce swelling
- Warm compresses thereafter to hasten resorption of hemorrhage

ORBITAL BLOWOUT FRACTURE

The most common locations for an orbital fracture caused by blunt trauma are the medial wall and the orbital floor.

Signs

- Bony defect of orbital rim, found by palpation
- Infraorbital hypesthesia (due to involvement of infraorbital canal). Ask the patient if he or she can feel an object as it touches the lower lid/orbital rim.

- Enophthalmos
- Periorbital emphysema. Air in lids gives the sensation of "Rice Krispy" lids, termed *crepitus,* which is caused by communication between the orbit and the periorbital sinuses.
- Diplopia may be caused by entrapment of the inferior rectus muscle. Disparity increases on upgaze. Diplopia may also be caused simply by swelling of the orbital contents. Perform forced duction testing to confirm entrapment.

Management

- Computed tomography (CT) scan of the orbit. Most facilities have protocols that include axial and coronal scans.
- A blowout fracture rarely requires immediate surgery. Indications for surgery include frank enophthalmos, loss of more than one-half of the floor, and persistent diplopia lasting longer than 14 days.
- Oral antibiotics (e.g., cephalexin or erythromycin, 250–500 mg PO qid for 10 days) along with a nasal decongestant (Afrin) nasal spray twice daily may be indicated when an orbital wall fracture involves one of the sinuses.
- Acute, severe vision loss due to a fracture of the orbital apex involving the optic nerve requires emergency surgical decompression.

IRIDOCYCLITIS

The diagnosis and treatment of iritis are discussed in Chapter 6.

HYPHEMA

The management of traumatic hyphema (blood in the anterior chamber) is still controversial. There is disagreement about the necessity for hospitalization, cycloplegia, patching, and antifibrinolytic agents (e.g., aminocaproic acid). When immediate surgical intervention is not indicated, the goal is to prevent rebleeding and complications related to high intraocular pressure (IOP) and blood staining of the cornea.

Management

- Strict bed rest for 5 days
- Head elevated with pillows
- Eye shield over involved eye
- Daily monitor of IOP (hand-held applanation tonometer works well)
- No aspirin or blood thinners
- 5% Homatropine 3 times a day
- 1% Prednisolone acetate every 2 hours, or as needed to control inflammation
- Topical beta blocker or other antiglaucoma medication, as needed to control IOP
- Oral aminocaproic acid 50–100 mg/kg every 4 hours up to a maximum of 30 g/day for adults*
- B-scan ultrasound to help rule out retinal detachment when view of fundus is limited
- Antiemetics (e.g., prochlorperazine [Compazine]) (as needed)

Indications for Surgery

- Total hyphema with IOP >50 mm Hg for 5 days
- IOP >35 mm Hg for 7 days
- Evidence of optic atrophy
- Blood staining of cornea (yellow granules in corneal stroma)
- Greater than 50% hyphema for 8–9 days

Remember that the possibility of traumatic glaucoma exists for years after the injury, so regular IOP checks should be scheduled.

IRIDOPLEGIA

Pupil paralysis may be transient or permanent. The sphincter may also be ruptured from blunt trauma. Treatment is not necessary.

---

*Patients on aminocaproic acid should be monitored for drug-induced systemic hypotension, nausea, and lightheadedness. It may be advisable to obtain a coagulation profile before starting therapy.

IRIDODIALYSIS

- Disinsertion of the iris from the ciliary body may require surgical intervention if diplopia, blur, or glare are problems.
- The patient should be monitored for traumatic glaucoma (even years later).

TRAUMATIC CATARACT

- Vossius' ring (circle of iris pigment on anterior lens surface)
- Anterior or posterior cortical opacities, anterior nodular plaques, and wedge-shaped opacities
- Treatment is cataract surgery if the opacity is visually significant, although this is an elective procedure.

LUXED/SUBLUXED CRYSTALLINE LENS

Rupture of zonules and subluxation may be evident after dilation or may be indicated by iridodonesis or phacodonesis (quivering iris or lens).

Treatment

- A ruptured lens may require prompt surgery to prevent phacoanaphylactic uveitis from leaking lens protein.
- Surgery can be delayed (sometimes indefinitely) for a posteriorly dislocated lens.
- For a lens that has been dislocated anteriorly into the anterior chamber, constrict the pupil with pilocarpine and initiate emergency surgery.
- Pupillary block glaucoma (the displaced lens blocks the pupil) can sometimes be relieved by the use of mydriatics, topical beta blockers, and systemic hyperosmotics. Laser iridotomy or surgery may also be necessary.
- Suspect Marfan's syndrome, syphilis, Marchesani's syndrome, or homocystinuria for subluxation with minor or no trauma.

SCLERAL RUPTURE

Globe rupture may be obvious, but on occasion other clinical findings in more subtle cases may lead to the correct diagnosis.

Signs and Symptoms

- Ocular hypotony (low IOP)
- Deepening or shallowing of the anterior chamber
- Intraocular hemorrhage
- Hemorrhagic chemosis
- Altered pupil shape

Management

- The patient and the examiner must take care not to put pressure on the globe to prevent extrusion of the intraocular contents.
- Bacterial and fungal cultures should be obtained if contamination is likely.
- Tetanus prophylaxis
- Intravenous antibiotics (e.g., vancomycin and ceftazadime)
- Protect eye with a shield.
- Make patient NPO (nothing to eat or drink).
- Surgical repair

VITREOUS HEMORRHAGE

Sources

- Retinal tear or detachment
- Rupture of ciliary body
- Retinal vessels (including neovascularization)

Management

- Rule out rupture of globe (see above).
- Examine for retinal tears or detachments.

- When the retina cannot be visualized, confrontation fields and ultrasonography are indicated to rule out detachment. The patient should be monitored until the hemorrhage clears.

BERLIN'S EDEMA

Retinal edema may produce reduced visual acuity and a cloudy swelling of the retina after blunt trauma. Treatment is not necessary since Berlin's edema usually subsides in several days to weeks, although a permanent visual defect is possible.

RETINAL TEARS AND DETACHMENTS

The diagnosis of traumatic retinal tears and detachments is made through visualization, but there are some characteristics not often seen in nontraumatic tears and detachments:

- Retinal dialysis from trauma occurs near the ora at the posterior border of the vitreous base.
- The superonasal and inferotemporal quadrants are most likely to be affected by dialysis.
- Traumatic retinal detachments are less bullous than nontraumatic detachments.
- Treatment is surgery as soon as possible.

RETROBULBAR HEMORRHAGE

Retrobulbar hemorrhage may occur in association with intraocular surgery (e.g., after block) or in association with trauma. Vision loss can be swift, requiring immediate intervention.

Signs and Symptoms

- Proptosis with resistance to retropulsion
- Significant subconjunctival hemorrhage
- Often with pain and decreased vision
- Eyelid ecchymosis
- May have increased IOP

- May demonstrate decreased ocular motility
- Pulsating central retinal artery may be observed and may indicate incipient retinal artery occlusion
- Choroidal folds may indicate incipient vision loss

Management (One or More of the Following)

- Lateral canthotomy and cantholysis for vision-threatening hemorrhage. Clamp lateral canthus for 1 minute with a hemostat. Make a horizontal 1-cm incision into the compressed tissue with sterile scissors. Cut the inferior arm of the lateral canthal tendon.
- Acetazolamide 500 mg PO
- 20% Mannitol 1–2 g/kg IV over 45 minutes
- Topical beta blocker (e.g., two drops 0.5% timolol) or apraclonidine 1% (Iopidine) (two drops)
- Orbital decompression for persistent ocular hypertension, impending or progressive vision loss, despite the above measures

TRAUMATIC OPTIC NEUROPATHY

Traumatic optic neuropathy typically occurs in association with deceleration injuries. It often occurs with the force of impact applied to the ipsilateral forehead or with midface trauma. Management is somewhat controversial. High-dose steroid recommendations are based on the National Acute Spinal Cord Injury Study 2, although there is no evidence that the results of this trial can be generalized to include optic nerve injuries.

Signs and Symptoms

- Usually immediately decreased vision—typically 20/400 or worse in the involved eye
- Delayed vision loss suggests an optic nerve sheath hematoma.
- Visual field loss
- Afferent pupillary defect
- The optic nerve may be normal in appearance or show swelling.

Management

- Treatment should be offered as soon as feasible.
- Obtain a CT scan of the head and orbits to rule out optic canal fracture or optic nerve sheath hematoma.
- Canthotomy or cantholysis if the orbit is tense.
- Drain subperiosteal hematoma if present.
- Methylprednisolone 30 mg/kg IV loading and 5.4 mg/kg per hour IV thereafter.
- Switch to prednisone PO with rapid taper after 48 hours if the patient is improving on IV steroids.
- Consider surgical decompression of the optic canal if the patient is deteriorating on drug tapering or shows no response to steroids.

OTHER BLUNT INJURIES

- Avulsion of the optic nerve usually results in very poor vision. Treatment is not necessary.
- Choroidal rupture can result in severe visual disability when it occurs through the macula. The patient should be monitored for development of a neovascular membrane (Amsler grid once per week, fundus examination at least yearly). Initially, treatment is not necessary.

CORNEAL ABRASION

- Elicit a detailed history from the patient. A high-speed foreign body may require a careful search for penetration and radiologic studies.
- Instill a topical anesthetic agent if needed for adequate examination.
- Evert lids to rule out a foreign body.
- Stain with fluorescein. Illustrate its size and location on a chart.

Treatment

1. Contact lens induced/from a tree branch, etc.
   - No pressure patch
   - If an infiltrate is present, it should be treated as a corneal ulcer. (See section on corneal ulcer in Chapter 5.)

- If there is no infiltrate, administer tobramycin or ofloxacin drops 4–6 times a day. Use ointment at bedtime.
- Instill cycloplegic (e.g., 2% cyclopentolate).
- Monitor daily until there is complete resolution.

2. Non–contact lens induced
- Instill cycloplegic (e.g., 2% cyclopentolate).
- Instill any antibiotic ointment.
- Use a pressure patch for large abrasion for 24 hours.
- Small abrasions (less than 20% of the total corneal area) can be treated with topical antibiotic ointments.
- Topical nonsteroidal drops (e.g., Ketorolac 0.5% qid) can assist with analgesia.
- See the patient in 24 hours. Repatch if necessary or prescribe antibiotic drops 4 times a day for 3 or 4 days.
- Consider hypertonic sodium chloride drops or ointment for persistent or recurrent erosions.

SUPERFICIAL FOREIGN BODIES

Always obtain the patient's history. High-speed foreign bodies require a careful examination, including dilation and possibly radiologic studies, to rule out or locate intraocular foreign bodies.

Management

- Instill a topical anesthetic agent (e.g., proparacaine).
- Remove the foreign body with a foreign body spud or other appropriate instrument. (Very superficial foreign bodies can occasionally be removed by irrigation. Forceps may be more appropriate for conjunctival foreign bodies.) Remove any superficial rust ring with an Alger brush/rust ring drill.
- Deeper rust may be left alone, especially if it is in the visual axis, to allow for migration to the surface and possible easier removal at a later date.
- A resulting epithelial defect should be managed as for corneal abrasion above (i.e., cycloplegic, antibiotic, pressure patch).

Note: For cases in which penetration is suspected, immediate hospitalization and surgery may be required. Pressure on the globe should be avoided. The patient should have no food or drink. Place a protective shield (not a pressure patch) over the eye for transport.

CHEMICAL INJURIES

Most chemical injuries to the eyes are relatively minor. Prompt attention is crucial for more severe chemical burns.

- Advise the patient to initiate prompt lavage of the eye even before coming in to the office.
- Continue lavage in the office or emergency room.
- Remove all particulate matter.
- Determine the nature of the chemical. Alkali burns (e.g., lime, ammonia) may continue to cause destruction for prolonged periods. Acid damage is more immediate.
- Litmus paper can be used to determine if lavage has been sufficient. Neutralizing agents are seldom effective.
- Alkali burns often cause pressure increases.
- Perforation may necessitate emergency surgery.
- Topical steroids are often indicated during the first few days to limit scarring and vascularization but can cause corneal melting and predispose to infection. They should be rapidly tapered after the first 1–2 weeks after an alkali burn in particular because of reports that they lead to corneal melts and other complications. They probably should be used if there is a significant anterior chamber reaction, in the face of significant inflammation or if membranes or symblepharon form.
- Other treatment measures include cycloplegics, topical antibiotics, and, in cases of secondary pressure increases, antiglaucoma drugs.
- Alkali burns may benefit from collagenase inhibitors such as acetylcysteine (Mucomyst) or perfusion with 0.024-M Na EDTA (dilute 0.5-M disodium edetate with 20 parts normal saline).
- Oral ascorbic acid (vitamin C), 2 g/day, may reduce the incidence of corneal ulceration.

LID LACERATIONS

Only uncomplicated lid lacerations should be repaired outside the operating room. Uncomplicated lacerations are those *not* involving the lacrimal apparatus or the levator aponeurosis or associated with other ocular injuries requiring intraocular surgery, such as an intraocular foreign body.

Management

- Tetanus prophylaxis
- Consider rabies prophylaxis for animal bites.
- Clean the area with povidone-iodine (Betadine).
- Do *not* shave eyebrows.
- Apply a local subcutaneous anesthetic agent.
- Irrigate the wound copiously.
- Remove foreign bodies in the wound.
- Consider delayed wound closure for contaminated wounds.
- After instilling a drop of proparacaine into the eye, apply a protective eye shell over the globe.
- Under sterile conditions, repair the laceration using a 6-0 silk suture (Fig. 2.1).
- If the lid margin is involved, it is generally closed first with three sutures. The first suture is placed through the gray line and the other two are placed anterior and posterior to the first.
- Leaving the sutures long allows them to be tucked into the first anterior suture. The first anterior suture is tied over the long suture ends of the lid margin sutures, preventing them from rubbing the cornea.
- Deep lacerations may require two-layered closure using 6-0 absorbable Vicryl suture.
- Apply bacitracin ointment.
- Systemic antibiotics (dicloxacillin 500 mg PO qid) are given for contaminated wounds. Oral penicillin is a good choice for bites.
- Superficial sutures can be removed in 4–6 days.
- Eyelid margin sutures are removed in 10–14 days.

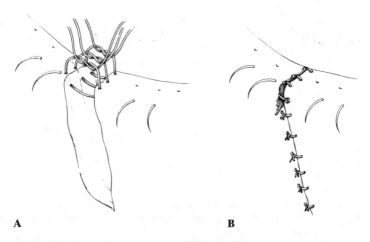

A   **B**

Fig. 2.1   A. Vertical eyelid laceration repair. The first suture is placed through the gray line. Any interruption of the margin is repaired first. B. After alignment of the margin, the skin is closed with interrupted sutures. (Reprinted with permission from F Newell. Ophthalmology Principles and Concepts [7th ed]. St. Louis: Mosby-Year Book, 1992.)

NOTES

3

Conjunctivitis

The diagnosis and treatment of a typical case of conjunctivitis, as presented to the primary care eye physician, remain an inexact science. Because of the very low morbidity associated with conjunctivitis, laboratory studies are usually reserved for unusual cases or those cases unresponsive to initial therapy.

KEY POINTS

- Verify that the inflammation is confined to the conjunctiva. This is confirmed by the observation that the injected vessels move with the conjunctiva or blanch with the use of topical phenylephrine.
- Pain and decreased visual acuity are *not* features consistent with the diagnosis of conjunctivitis. The presence of these symptoms should cause the clinician to rethink the diagnosis.
- More serious red eye etiologies, such as corneal ulcers and acute glaucoma, can likewise be ruled out by careful slit-lamp biomicroscopy and intraocular pressure measurements.
- One of the most common reasons for therapeutic failure is incorrect initial diagnosis. If the clinician is willing to accept not achieving 100% accuracy using only clinical clues to diagnose conjunctivitis, he or she stands a much greater chance of achieving eventual success.
- Initial therapeutic decisions are based on history and clinical clues. Laboratory studies (e.g., smears, cultures, sensitivities) should be ordered whenever the reason for therapeutic failure is not obvious. Tables 3.1 and 3.2 can be consulted to help establish a working diagnosis.

Table 3.1 Differential Diagnosis of Common Forms of Conjunctivitis

Clinical Feature	Bacterial	Viral	Allergic	Chlamydial
Exudate	Purulent or mucopurulent	Watery	Mucoid (white and stringy)	Scant mucopurulent
Papillae[a]	Usually present	Absent	Present	Usually present
Follicles[b]	Usually absent	Present	Absent	Present
Pseudomembrane	Rare	Occasional	Absent	Absent
Fever/sore throat	Rare	Common	No association	No association
Preauricular node	Infrequent	Common	Absent	Common
Quick smear characteristics	PMNs	Monocytes, lymphocytes	May show eosinophils	PMNs, lymphocytes, cytoplasmic inclusions
Giemsa/Diff-				

PMNs = polymorphonuclear leukocytes.
[a]Papillae appear as polygonal conjunctival elevations with a central vascular stalk.
[b]Follicles appear as translucent round elevations of the conjunctiva.

Table 3.2 Differential Diagnosis of Chronic Forms of Conjunctivitis

Disorder	Key Characteristics	Management
Dry eye	Stain with rose bengal; involves exposed cornea; reduced Schirmer's	Ocular lubricants; patching; punctal occlusion
Adult inclusion conjunctivitis	Usually in sexually active adolescents and young adults; follicular; peripheral or superior keratitis	Tetracycline 1–2 g/day; erythromycin 1.0–1.5 g in 4 divided doses; or doxycycline 100 mg twice daily for 3 wks
Rosacea	Associated with facial eruption	Oral tetracycline; lid scrubs
Blepharitis	Thickened lid margins; crusting; collarettes of lashes; madarosis	Lid hygiene; topical antibiotic ointment
Medicamentosa	Associated with prolonged use of topical ophthalmics	Discontinue offending agents
Angular conjunctivitis	Maceration of tissue at lateral canthus caused by *Staphylococcus* or *Moraxella*	Topical antibiotics
Pemphigoid	Older patients; progressive conjunctival erosions; fibrosis; symblepharon	Oral prednisone; dapsone; immunosuppressants; ocular lubricants
Parinaud's syndrome	Associated lymphadenopathy; exposure to cats, rabbits, etc.	Erythromycin, azithromycin, or ciprofloxacin for cat scratch; streptomycin for tularemia; KI for sporotrichosis; specific therapy for syphilis and tuberculosis

KI = potassium iodide.

BACTERIAL CONJUNCTIVITIS

Bacterial conjunctivitis is one of the more common causes of red eye that requires the assistance of an eye physician. Generally, bacterial conjunctivitis can be categorized as acute, hyperacute, or chronic.

Acute Bacterial Conjunctivitis

Clinical Features

- Conjunctival injection (redness) usually accompanied by a muco-purulent discharge.
- Patients often complain of the lids sticking together in the morning.
- Often there is a fine, velvety papillary reaction of the palpebral conjunctiva.
- A mild superficial keratitis is not uncommon.

Management

- Bacterial conjunctivitis is most often treated without knowledge of the etiologic organism. Instead, a broad-spectrum antimicrobial agent such as trimethoprim and polymyxin B (Polytrim) or a triple antibiotic such as neomycin, polymyxin B, and gramicidin is prescribed as an eyedrop to be used 4–6 times a day (consult Table 22.1 for more information).
- An antimicrobial ointment may also be used at night.
- If no clinical improvement is noted within 5 days, the clinician should rethink the diagnosis and consider appropriate laboratory studies.

Hyperacute Bacterial Conjunctivitis

Clinical Features

- Patients often present with an acutely red eye with a large amount of purulent discharge. This is much more severe than the more common acute bacterial conjunctivitis.

- In contrast to acute bacterial conjunctivitis, the patient with hyper-acute bacterial conjunctivitis may complain of pain and show prominent preauricular adenopathy.

Etiology

- Gonococcus (from infected genitalia)
- Meningococcus
- *Haemophilus*
- Streptococcus
- *Corynebacterium diphtheriae*

Management

- Because the etiologic agent is most often *Neisseria gonorrhoeae,* an organism that can penetrate intact epithelium, hyperacute conjunctivitis is approached with much more gravity and urgency than simple acute conjunctivitis.
- Smears for Gram staining should be collected and processed as soon as possible to identify the characteristic gram-negative diplococci.
- Thayer-Martin and chocolate agar plates for anaerobic cultures should be used.
- Systemic antibiotics as well as topical therapy (ceftriaxone, 1 g IM). For penicillin-allergic patients, spectinomycin (2 g IM), ciprofloxacin (500 mg PO bid for 5 days), or ofloxacin (400 mg PO for 5 days) can be substituted.
- Corneal ulceration requires hospitalization and treatment with ceftriaxone, 1 g IV q12h.
- Topical ciprofloxacin, ofloxacin, erythromycin, or bacitracin may also be used.

Chronic Bacterial Conjunctivitis/Blepharitis

Clinical Appearance

- The patient may show low-grade conjunctivitis with madarosis (loss of lashes) and thickened hyperemic lid margins.

- Often there is a history of recurrent hordeolum.
- Early morning matting of the lids may be a symptom.
- Discharge is usually minimal.

Management

- The patient should be instructed to perform lid scrubs followed by the application of an antibiotic ointment such as polymyxin B and bacitracin to the lid margins twice a day for 1 week.
- Thereafter a maintenance regimen of once-a-day lid scrubs can often prevent recurrences.
- Bacterial cultures should be performed for resistant cases.

Laboratory for Bacterial Conjunctivitis

- Make sure antibiotic therapy has been discontinued for at least 24 hours.
- Culturette, which is commercially available, is an acceptable method to obtain conjunctival cultures in most cases.
- Alternatively, one may wipe a sterile cotton-tipped applicator, moistened with nonpreserved sterile saline or sterile broth, on the palpebral conjunctiva or lower fornix. The applicator can then be swabbed directly on a sheep blood and chocolate agar plate. Similarly, using sterile technique, a swab can be broken off into a vial of thioglycolate broth.
- In unilateral cases, a culture should also be taken from the fellow eye, as a control.
- Ask for bacterial cultures and a sensitivity test.
- Provide the laboratory with a list of available topical ophthalmic antibacterial agents.
- Do not forget that anaerobic transport is necessary for *Neisseria* (hyperacute conjunctivitis). Ask a laboratory technician how culture transport should be accomplished if *Neisseria* is suspected.
- It is a good idea to obtain conjunctival smears also at this time. After instilling a topical anesthetic agent, a platinum spatula is scraped across the palpebral conjunctiva. This specimen can then be smeared

on a clean microscopic slide. Request a Giemsa or Diff-Quick stain to identify the type of inflammatory cells (see Table 3.1).

NEONATAL CONJUNCTIVITIS (OPHTHALMIA NEONATORUM)

Conjunctivitis in infants is a special situation requiring investigation into the etiology and more intensive therapy. The mother's history and circumstances of the delivery are obviously relevant to management. The age of the newborn at the time he or she contracts conjunctivitis can be very helpful in determining the etiology.

Chemical conjunctivitis (from Credé prophylaxis)	days 1–2
Chlamydia	days 5–12
Nasolacrimal obstruction	day 1
Other bacteria	days 3–30

Management

- Prepare a Gram stain of the conjunctival scraping to look for the gram-negative intracellular diplococci of gonococcus.
- Prepare a Giemsa stain of the conjunctival scraping to look for the cytoplasmic inclusions found in chlamydial infection.
- Conjunctival culture on blood agar, chocolate, and Thayer-Martin media
- Perform a chlamydial culture or antibody tests (Microtrak).
- Treat gonococcal infection with ceftriaxone 125 mg IM for 1–2 days. Irrigate with sterile saline solution and topical bacitracin ointment, tetracycline, or penicillin G drops (100,000 U/ml) every 2 hours for the first 2 or 3 days, then 5 times a day for 7 days. Examine the patient for systemic infections (take blood and cerebrospinal fluid cultures). These infections may require more intensive therapy for longer periods.
- Treat *Haemophilus influenzae* with ampicillin 50–200 mg/kg IM or IV every 12 hours for 10 days. Topical antibiotics such as gentamicin and ciprofloxacin should also be used. Chloramphenicol is indicated in ampicillin-resistant cases.

Treat chlamydial infections with oral erythromycin, 50 mg/kg per day in 4 divided doses plus topical sulfonamide or erythromycin 4 times a day for 3 weeks.

ADENOVIRAL KERATOCONJUNCTIVITIS

A number of different serotypes of adenovirus are known to cause ocular syndromes that may be indistinguishable from each other during the early stages of disease. The hallmark feature is an acute follicular reaction of the palpebral conjunctiva. Many patients will present with preauricular lymphadenopathy. The incubation period is generally 5–10 days but may last up to 21 days. Viral shedding may persist for another 7–12 days.

Viral Ocular Syndromes

Acute Follicular Conjunctivitis

Clinically, acute follicular conjunctivitis is usually confined to one eye. A mild epithelial keratitis may be present, but there are no stromal infiltrates. There is usually a rapid resolution of symptoms within just a few days.

Pharyngoconjunctival Fever

Pharyngoconjunctival fever is often seen in children and is characterized by fever, headache, and upper respiratory symptoms (e.g., sore throat, cough). Occasionally, it may be associated with head cold, cough, loss of appetite, nausea, and muscle aches. It may be bilateral or unilateral. Keratitis is usually mild without stromal infiltrates.

Epidemic Keratoconjunctivitis

Up to one-half of patients may show pharyngitis and rhinitis (sore throat, runny nose). Hyperemia and chemosis of the conjunctiva is common. Occasionally, hemorrhages are present. Patients commonly show membranes or pseudomembranes. Within 3 days of onset, diffuse punctate erosions may develop. Course granular subepithelial infiltrates may appear from 6 to 12 days and persist for months. Iritis is rare.

Management of Viral Conjunctivitis

Patient education is an important part of management. Because there is no cure for this disorder, the disease must run its course (analogous to the common cold). Management is aimed at improving comfort and preventing transmission.

* Topical decongestants and eye washes
* Removal of symptomatic membranes with forceps or cotton swab
* In severe cases, topical steroids for patient comfort or when infiltrates significantly affect vision. Note: Infiltrates often return when medication is discontinued and may persist for a year or longer.
* Caution against sharing towels or contact with other people. School children and health care professionals should be quarantined.
* Hand washing by the physician and patient
* Sterilization of instruments

CHLAMYDIAL KERATOCONJUNCTIVITIS

The chlamydial organism is responsible for three separate clinical entities: (1) neonatal inclusion conjunctivitis (in the newborn), (2) adult inclusion conjunctivitis (in sexually active adolescents and adults), and (3) trachoma (in underdeveloped countries and among the American Indian population).

Adult inclusion conjunctivitis is the disorder seen most commonly in clinical practice and is discussed in this section.

Clinical Signs

* Chronic follicular conjunctivitis
* Mucopurulent discharge
* Punctate keratitis and/or micropannus

Laboratory

- Giemsa stain: polys and monocytes. Cytoplasmic inclusions are rarely seen in adult inclusion conjunctivitis.
- Fluorescent antibody stain (Microtrak) of conjunctival smears
- Chlamydial culture

Management

- Oral tetracycline, 250 mg qid, or doxycycline, 100 mg bid, for 3 weeks, *or*
- Oral erythromycin for women who are pregnant or nursing, children under age 8 years, and patients who are intolerant of tetracycline
- A one-time dose of azithromycin 1 g PO has been reported to be an acceptable alternative.
- Topical tetracycline or erythromycin 4–6 times a day
- Treatment for sexual partners
- Consultation and treatment for other venereal diseases

ALLERGIC CONJUNCTIVITIS

Allergic reactions are adverse reactions of the immune system, which result in damage to the host. Ocular allergies generally fall into one of two broad categories: immediate hypersensitivity (type I) and delayed hypersensitivity (type IV).

Immediate Hypersensitivity

An immediate hypersensitivity allergic reaction is mediated by histamine and requires previous exposure to the antigen. Examples include:

- Hay fever conjunctivitis
- Chronic atopic conjunctivitis
- Vernal conjunctivitis
- Giant papillary conjunctivitis

Vernal Conjunctivitis

A conjunctivitis that is most prevalent in young men with an onset at about puberty. There is often a hereditary predisposition.

Signs and Symptoms
- Conjunctival cobblestones over the upper tarsal plate
- Copious, highly elastic, cordlike mucus
- Little or no significant conjunctival hyperemia
- Trantas' dots (raised white superficial infiltrates at the limbus)
- Gelatinous, translucent, globular deposits at the limbus
- Diffuse keratitis in severe cases
- Shield ulcer (a central epithelial defect with overlying white plaque)
- Intense itching, photophobia, and pain
- Eosinophils on scrapings
- Pseudomembrane

Management
Depending on severity, a combination of several of the measures listed below may be necessary.
- Identification of allergens and elimination or avoidance
- Air conditioning with filters
- Glasses or goggles to limit exposure to airborne allergens
- Limit eye rubbing.
- Tear substitutes
- Vasoconstrictors
- Topical antihistamines (e.g., levocabastine)
- Cold compresses
- Aspirin in recalcitrant cases (up to 2,400 mg per day in four divided doses)*
- Pulse therapy of a topical steroid (e.g., rimexolone 1% applied six to eight times per day for 1 week, followed by rapid tapering for severe cases to bring the inflammation under control)

---

*Where ulceration of the gastrointestinal mucosa is present, and its effect on platelets is evident, caution must be used when aspirin is prescribed at such doses.

- Patching with antibiotic-steroid combinations is effective for shield ulcers
- Cromolyn sodium 4% or lodoxamide 0.1%: instill 1–2 drops four times per day to decrease or eliminate the need for steroids

Seasonal Allergic Conjunctivitis

Seasonal allergic conjunctivitis often is found in allergic individuals who have seasonal exacerbations. Often it is associated with systemic hay fever. Individuals may be sensitive to grasses, hay, weeds, or tree pollens.

Signs and Symptoms
- Itching
- Tearing, burning
- Conjunctival chemosis, hyperemia, papillae
- Often with a clear discharge

Treatment
- Avoid exposure
- 0.1% lodoxamide tromethamine (Alomide) or 4% cromolyn sodium, 1 drop four times a day, starting before the season begins
- Systemic antihistamines (e.g., oral terfenadine, 60 mg two times per day, or astemizole, 10 mg three times per day)
- Short-term topical steroids for severe exacerbations
- Topical nonsteroidals (e.g., 0.5% ketorolac, 1 drop four times per day)
- Desensitization for disabling allergy

Giant Papillary Disorders of the Conjunctiva

Giant capillary conjunctivitis (GPC) is a disorder characterized by the eruption of giant papillae on the upper palpebral conjunctiva as a result of chronic trauma from contact lenses, suture barbs, ocular prostheses, or other foreign bodies.

Signs and Symptoms
- The hallmark feature is giant cobblestone papillae of the superior palpebral conjunctiva.

- Itching, tearing, mucus discharge
- Recognizable foreign body on or in the eye (e.g., contact lens, suture barb)
- In cases of contact lens wearers, there is often a complaint of excessive lens movement and lens deposition.

Treatment
- Discontinue lens wear or remove offending foreign body.
- Frequent use of enzymes for lenses; change sterilization technique
- Consider switch to disposable contact lenses or gas-permeable lenses.
- 0.1% lodoxamide tromethamine (Alomide), 1 drop four times per day

Atopic Keratoconjunctivitis

An ocular inflammatory condition appearing in teenagers and young adults. Patients generally have a history of eczema, systemic atopic rhinitis, asthma, or atopic dermatitis.

Signs and Symptoms
- Thickened erythematous lid skin and margins
- Cicatrization and symblepharon formation
- Corneal vascularization
- Cataracts in 10% of patients (anterior or posterior subcapsular)
- Kerataconus
- Susceptible to herpes simplex, blepharitis, or keratitis
- Staphylococcal infections are common.

Treatment
- Systemic antihistamines (e.g., oral terfenadine, 60 mg two times per day, or oral astemizole, 10 mg three times per day)
- Instill one drop 0.1% lodoxamide tromethamine (Alomide) or 4% cromolyn sodium four times per day.
- Brief course of treatment with steroids for acute exacerbations
- Instill 2% cyclosporin A drops four times per day for severe cases
- Treat associated infections.

Delayed Hypersensitivity

Delayed hypersensitivity reactions do not involve antibodies or histamine, but rather sensitized lymphocytes. The reaction takes 24–72 hours to become maximal. Examples include:

- Contact dermatoconjunctivitis: common offenders are neomycin, gentamicin, and cosmetics
- Phlyctenulosis: small, pinkish-white nodules near the limbus or on the cornea. They represent a hypersensitivity to *Staphylococcus* or tuberculosis.

Treatment

- Avoidance of antigen. Lid scrubs and antibiotics for *Staphylococcus phlyctenulosis*. Tuberculosis workup if this is suspected. Discontinue offending medication or cosmetic.
- Cold compresses, eye washes
- Instill topical corticosteroids (e.g., 0.1% fluorometholone, 1 drop four times per day) if necessary.

KERATITIS SICCA (DRY EYES)

Tear layer instability/insufficiency is one of the most common causes of chronic ocular irritation and keratoconjunctivitis.

Associated Signs and Symptoms

- Burning and foreign body sensation
- Visual blurring that may clear on blinking
- Contact lens intolerance
- Corneal staining with rose bengal and/or fluorescein
- Decreased tear breakup time (<10 seconds)
- Mucus or debris in tear film
- Epiphora (watery eyes) as a result of ocular irritation, which is often seen in association with wind, reading, watching television, air conditioning, etc.
- Reduced Schirmer's tear test (<10 mm of wetting after 5 minutes)

Associated Conditions

- Collagen vascular disease (e.g., rheumatoid arthritis, Sjögren's disease, lupus)
- Antihistamines, oral contraceptives, and other medications
- Conjunctival scarring
- Idiopathic

Treatment

Treatment is generally stepwise, with more severe cases requiring greater levels of intervention. In any case, aggravating conditions (e.g., certain medications, blepharitis) should be eliminated.

Level 1

- Artificial tears 3–6 times a day

Level 2

- Preservative-free artificial tears every 1–2 hours, or carboxymethylcellulose (Celluvisc) every 2–4 hours during the day
- Bland ophthalmic ointment (e.g., Lacri-Lube) at night

Level 3

- Bland ophthalmic ointment every 4–6 hours with artificial tears as needed
- Consider patching (at bedtime or during the day).
- Consider Lacrisert (tear insert).
- Punctal or canalicular occlusion (temporary occlusion with dissolvable collagen rods is recommended as a trial before permanent occlusion)

Level 4

- Lateral tarsorrhaphy

PINGUECULA/PTERYGIUM

Pingueculae and pterygia are both yellow-white elevations on the anterior eye surface. The etiology of both may be related to exposure to sunlight, dust, wind, and drying.

- Both tend to be more common nasally.
- Pingueculae are confined to the conjunctiva.
- Pterygia extend onto the cornea. They are typically horizontally oriented and triangular in shape, with the apex directed toward the central cornea.
- Pterygia may originate from pingueculae.

Treatment

- Ocular lubricants and/or mild vasoconstrictors for comfort
- Short-term topical steroids (e.g., fluorometholone qid for 4–5 days) for more severe inflammation
- Protection from sun and wind by the use of sunglasses or eyeglasses with ultraviolet coatings
- Growing pterygia should be surgically excised.
- The application of beta radiation, mitomycin, or conjunctival transplant may prevent regrowth.
- Pingueculae rarely require surgical intervention.

PARINAUD'S OCULOGLANDULAR CONJUNCTIVITIS

Parinaud's oculoglandular conjunctivitis is the descriptive term for conjunctivitis associated with:

- Granulomas of the conjunctiva
- Ipsilateral swelling of preauricular and/or submandibular nodes
- Fever or rash (sometimes)

Etiology

- Cat scratch disease (Ask about contact with outdoor cats.)
- Tularemia (Hunters are at highest risk. Ask about outdoor activities and contact with rabbits.)
- Tuberculosis (Ask about contacts, cough, etc.)
- Syphilis (Ask about high-risk behavior, previous venereal diseases, and genital lesions.)

- Sarcoidosis (Prevalence is highest in black people.)
- Lymphoma or leukemia

Workup

- Conjunctival biopsy with Gram, Giemsa, and acid-fast stains
- Culture on blood, thioglycolate, Sabouraud's, and Löwenstein-Jensen media
- Complete blood cell count
- Rapid plasma reagin (RPR) and fluorescent treponemal antibody absorption (FTA-ABS) test if syphilis is possible
- Purified protein derivative for tuberculosis with mumps or candidal control
- Chest x-ray for sarcoid and tuberculosis
- Serologic titers for tularemia if suspected

Management

- Cat scratch disease: erythromycin, azithromycin, or ciprofloxacin orally plus topical gentamicin or polymyxin B/bacitracin for 2 weeks
- Tularemia: refer to internist; streptomycin 1 g/day IM for 7 days, plus 1 drop of gentamicin every 2 hours for 1 week, then every 4 hours until resolved
- Syphilis: refer to internist; systemic penicillin plus tetracycline ophthalmic ointment qid
- Tuberculosis: refer to internist for systemic treatment
- Lymphoma and leukemia: refer to oncologist

OCULAR ROSACEA

Rosacea is a dermatologic condition associated with hyperplasia of the sebaceous glands. It generally affects middle-aged adults. It can cause chronic conjunctivitis.

Signs and Symptoms

- Bilateral conjunctivitis
- Telangiectasia and erythema of the face
- Pustules and papules on the face, chest, and back
- Rhinophyma
- Blepharitis and chalazia are common.
- Possible punctate keratitis and corneal vascularization
- Marginal infiltrates not uncommon
- Rarely corneal perforation
- Often foreign body sensation or burning

Treatment

- Oral antibiotics: tetracycline or erythromycin, 250 mg qid with slow tapering off after 4–6 weeks, and possibly low-dose maintenance (i.e., 250 mg/day)
- Ocular lubricants for comfort
- Lid scrubs and hot compresses
- Antibiotic ointment (e.g., bacitracin) to lid margins twice a day for concurrent bacterial blepharitis

OCULAR PEMPHIGOID

Ocular pemphigoid is an uncommon but often missed cause of chronic conjunctivitis. Pemphigoid is a chronic inflammatory disease of the mucous membranes and tends to affect older individuals (age >55 years).

Signs and Symptoms

- Bilateral chronic conjunctivitis with remissions and exacerbations
- Inferior symblepharon (foreshortening of the lower fornix with adhesion of palpebral to ocular conjunctiva)
- Poor tear film
- Possible vesicles and bullae of other mucous membranes and skin

- Possible punctate keratitis, corneal ulcers, corneal neovascularization, entropion, trichiasis, and limited eye movement secondary to symblepharon

Treatment

- Ocular lubricants including artificial tears and ointments
- Short-term topical steroids (e.g., fluorometholone 0.1% qid for 4–5 days) for more severe inflammation
- Lid hygiene and treatment of any blepharitis or secondary bacterial infections
- Systemic steroids (prednisone) and/or immunosuppressive drugs (e.g., dapsone, cyclophosphamide) may be of benefit for severe, progressive cases.
- Protection from wind and drying by the use of sunglasses, eyeglasses, or goggles
- Possibly oculoplastic surgery for advanced cases

FLOPPY EYELID SYNDROME

Spontaneous eversion of the eyelids with rubbing of the exposed palpebral conjunctiva on pillows or sheets can result in chronic conjunctivitis.

Signs and Symptoms

- Conjunctival injection with mucoid discharge
- Patients often obese
- Easily everted upper eyelid
- Superior tarsal papillary conjunctivitis
- Superficial punctate keratitis not uncommon

Treatment

- Ocular lubricants
- Eye shield over affected eye at night
- Discourage patient from sleeping on stomach.
- Surgical correction for select cases

PHTHIRIASIS PALPEBRARUM

Phthiriasis palpebrarum refers to eyelid infestation with *Phthirus pubis*, the crab louse. This louse normally inhabits the pubic or inguinal regions. It can be transferred via sexual contact or by contaminated towels or bedding.

Signs and Symptoms

- Itching
- Adult lice and nits (eggs) at the base of lashes
- Dark red, crusty fecal material on the lid margins

Management

- Remove adult lice with forceps using the slit lamp.
- Epilate lashes with nits.
- A bland ophthalmic ointment applied twice a day to the lid margin for 10 to 14 days can be used to smother the parasites.
- 0.25% physostigmine ointment applied twice a day has been recommended, but its use is limited by undesirable side effects (e.g., miosis, brow ache).
- Treatment of body and pubic hair with a pediculicide (e.g., gamma benzene hexachloride [Kwell] or a pyrethrin product [RID]).
- Wash bedding and clothes in hottest temperature available.
- Consider investigation for other sexually transmitted diseases.

SUPERIOR LIMBIC KERATOCONJUNCTIVITIS

Superior limbic keratoconjunctivitis (SLK) is a chronic, recurrent condition most commonly affecting women between the ages of 20 to 70 years. Unless specifically looked for, it is often misdiagnosed. A form of this disorder appears in contact lens wearers.

Signs and Symptoms

- Symptoms often include burning and the feeling of a foreign body.
- Usually bilateral

- Fine papillary reaction on the superior conjunctiva
- Injection and thickening of the superior bulbar conjunctiva
- Fine rose bengal staining of the superior bulbar conjunctiva and cornea
- Superior filamentary keratitis

Management

- Discontinue contact lens wear in contact lens patients.
- A significant number of patients have thyroid dysfunction. If not already diagnosed, order thyroid function tests.
- Try topical lubricants in mild cases.
- Some success has been reported with use of a bandage soft contact lens.
- Chemical cauterization of superior bulbar and superior tarsal conjunctiva with 0.5–1.0% silver nitrate solution (from wax ampules)
- Thermal cauterization of the superior bulbar or tarsal conjunctiva (with laser or cautery)
- Surgical resection of the superior bulbar conjunctiva

STEVENS-JOHNSON SYNDROME (ERYTHEMA MULTIFORME MAJUS)

An acute inflammatory vesiculobullous reaction of the skin and mucous membranes. Erythema multiforme minor refers to involvement of the skin with sparing of mucous membranes. The mortality from intercurrent infections in erythema multiforme majus is 20%.

Common Inciting Agents

- Sulfonamides
- Anticonvulsants
- Salicylates
- Penicillin
- Ampicillin
- Isoniazid
- Herpes simplex

- Streptococci
- Adenovirus
- Mycoplasma

Signs and Symptoms

- Often presents as a febrile illness with cough, headache, and malaise
- Skin eruption may follow in a few days with target lesions (red center, surrounded by a pale ring, and then a red ring).
- Maculopapular or bullous skin lesions may also appear.
- Mucous membranes may be affected by bullous lesions with membranes or pseudomembranes.
- Late complications include conjunctival shrinkage, mucin tear deficiency, and trichiasis.

Management

- The systemic condition may require systemic corticosteroids.
- Ocular lubrication with artificial tears and ointments
- The use of topical steroids is controversial.
- Daily lysis of symblepharon with glass rods or other instruments is advocated by some.
- Symblepharon rings also have been used.
- Treatment of ocular infections
- Surgical correction of entropion, trichiasis, etc. should not be performed until the disease is quiescent.

NOTES

4

Lids, Orbit, and Lacrimal Apparatus

DACRYOCYSTITIS

Dacryocystitis is an infection of the lacrimal drainage apparatus and is a cause of acquired epiphora. It may follow obstruction of the nasolacrimal duct.

Symptoms

- Epiphora (tearing)
- Pain, swelling, and redness over the lacrimal sac
- A mucoid discharge that can be expressed from the punctum by applying pressure over the lacrimal sac

Management

- Take smears and cultures of material expressed from the sac, including anaerobic and fungal.
- Attempt to decompress the sac by careful, gentle probing with Bowman 0 or 00 probe, followed by irrigation with topical antibiotic or antibiotic-steroid combination (e.g., tetracycline, trimethoprim/sulfamethoxazole).
- Instruct the patient to massage over the lacrimal sac while applying pressure over the lower lid to occlude the canaliculus (four times a day).
- Topical antibiotic (e.g., trimethoprim/sulfamethoxazole 4–6 times a day)
- Oral dicloxacillin or cephalexin 1–2 g in 4 divided doses for 10–14 days
- Switch antibiotics if cultures or sensitivities indicate.

- Warm compresses may be used if there is little inflammation, but they may promote fistula formation if there is an active infection.
- Incision and drainage of localized abscesses should be performed. The incised abscess is packed open and allowed to heal.
- Consider a computed tomographic (CT) scan in unresponsive, atypical cases.
- Febrile patients should be hospitalized and treated with intravenous antibiotics.
- Surgical correction of the occluded lacrimal apparatus is commonly required after resolution of the infection.

CHALAZION/HORDEOLUM

A *hordeolum* is a focal, acute infection within the eyelid glands and is characterized by:

- Pain and tenderness
- Focal lid swelling
- Blocked gland orifice

A *chalazion* is a chronic granuloma of meibomian glands.

- Focal mass within substance of eyelid
- Initial tenderness followed by little or no tenderness
- Chronic chalazia can be associated with hypercholesterolemia.

Both conditions are often associated with chronic lid conditions such as blepharitis and rosacea.

Treatment

- Hot compresses for 10 minutes 4 times a day
- Oral antibiotic if hordeolum is associated with preauricular adenopathy
- Lid hygiene (lid scrubs twice daily)
- Topical antibiotics if associated staphylococcal blepharitis or drainage occurs
- Curettage and excision or steroid injection of recalcitrant cases

Note: Sebaceous cell carcinoma should be suspected in recurrent chalazia.

PRESEPTAL CELLULITIS

Inflammation or infection of structures anterior to the orbital septum characterizes preseptal cellulitis. Orbital cellulitis is associated with proptosis, decreased vision, ocular motility disturbances, and fever. Both preseptal cellulitis and orbital cellulitis should be differentiated from allergic edema (itching with suggestive history) and chalazion (focal eyelid inflammation usually with palpable mass). Either condition may be the result of extension from a sinus infection or previous trauma.

Signs and Symptoms

- Erythema, edema, and warmth of eyelid
- Tenderness of lids
- Possible extension into the cheeks in children

Management

- Rule out orbital cellulitis (Table 4.1)—i.e., check visual acuity, pupil reaction, ocular motilities, proptosis, and significant fever.
- Prepare Gram stain and culture of open wounds.

Table 4.1   Orbital vs. Preseptal Cellulitis

	Preseptal Cellulitis	*Orbital Cellulitis*
Lid swelling, erythema	Present	Present
Decreased vision	Absent	Common
Double vision	Absent	Common
Proptosis	Absent	Common
Decreased sensation in V_1	Absent	Common
Retinal venous congestion and/or optic disc edema	Absent	Common
Fever	None or low grade	Common

- Obtain a CT scan for cases associated with trauma, or for confirmation of sinusitis, suspicion of foreign body, abscess, cavernous sinus thrombosis, or malignancy.
- Use oral antibiotics—e.g., dicloxacillin 250–500 mg PO q6h, amoxicillin/clavulanate (Augmentin) 250–500 mg PO q8h, cefaclor (Ceclor) 250–500 mg PO q8h, or erythromycin 250–500 mg PO q6h in adults.
- Hospitalization and IV antibiotics for young children, severe cases, and nonresponsive cases. Oxacillin 150 mg/kg/day in 6 divided doses for children, or 1–2 g q4h in adults, plus ceftazidime 30–50 mg/kg q8h in children (maximum, 6 g/day), or 1–2 g q8h in adults.
- Use hot compresses 4 times a day.
- Perform incision and drainage of abscesses, exploration and debridement of wounds with drain, and Gram stain and culture of drainage.
- Tetanus toxoid for cases associated with trauma and no recent immunization

ORBITAL CELLULITIS

Orbital cellulitis is a term applied to soft-tissue infection posterior to the orbital septum. It is associated with proptosis, chemosis, decreased vision, ocular motility disturbances, and fever. In 90% of cases, it results from extension of a sinus infection. It requires aggressive management because it may progress to cavernous sinus thrombosis, brain abscess, and death. See Table 4.1 for the differential diagnosis from preseptal cellulitis.

Signs and Symptoms

- Erythema, conjunctival chemosis
- Proptosis
- Restricted ocular motilities, often with pain
- Fever
- Often occurs with sinusitis on CT scan

- Decreased vision and/or pupillary involvement suggests orbital apex involved.

Management

- Hospitalize the patient.
- Complete blood count with differential
- Gram stain and culture of open wounds; blood cultures
- CT scan of orbits and sinuses. Rule out cavernous sinus involvement.
- IV antibiotics. Good initial choices include ampicillin/sulbactam (Unasyn) 1.5–3.0 g IV q6h, or vancomycin 1 g IV q12h (adjust for renal failure), ceftriaxone 1–2 g q12–24h, and metronidazole 15 mg/kg IV load, then 7.5 mg/kg q6h. For children, vancomycin 20 mg/kg IV q12h (adjust for renal failure) and ceftriaxone 50 mg/kg IV q12h is a good starting combination pending culture results.
- Ear, nose, and throat consult for any associated sinusitis
- Nasal decongestants for sinus involvement to promote drainage
- Incision and drainage of abscesses, exploration and debridement of wounds with a drain, and Gram stain and culture of drainage
- Tetanus toxoid for cases associated with trauma and no recent immunization

ORBITAL INFLAMMATORY SYNDROME (ORBITAL PSEUDOTUMOR)

Orbital inflammatory syndrome (OIS), or orbital pseudotumor, refers to an idiopathic inflammation of orbital tissues unrelated to thyroid ophthalmopathy, infection, or systemic disease. There are several different variants depending on the particular structures involved. These variants include dacryoadenitis (lacrimal gland involvement), myositis (extraocular muscle involvement), sclerotenonitis, or diffuse orbital involvement. Spread of inflammation to the orbital apex and cavernous sinus leads to the Tolosa-Hunt syndrome and painful ophthalmoplegia.

OIS in children is more likely to be bilateral (one-third of cases) and more likely to be associated with systemic findings such as headache, fever, lethargy, abdominal pain, and vomiting.

Signs and Symptoms

- Eyelid erythema, conjunctival injection, and chemosis
- Proptosis
- Restricted ocular motilities
- Orbital pain
- Decreased vision if the optic nerve or posterior sclera is involved
- Fever may be present.
- May show leukocytosis, elevated erythrocyte sedimentation rate, peripheral blood eosinophilia, and/or a positive antinuclear antibody (ANA) test

Management

- An orbital CT scan should be obtained. Involvement of the extraocular muscles typically results in thickening of the muscle and tendon in contrast to muscle-only involvement in thyroid ophthalmopathy.
- Work up bilateral cases for systemic vasculitis (e.g., systemic lupus erythematosus, polyarteritis nodosa, Wegener's granulomatosis).
- Initial therapy is generally with systemic steroids.
- Unresponsive cases may require biopsy confirmation of the diagnosis.
- Orbital irradiation and/or cyclophosphamide may be necessary in some patients (Fig. 4.1).

EYELID TUMORS

Diagnosis of eyelid tumors by inspection alone is highly inaccurate. Malignant tumors can mimic benign lesions. There are many cases of basal cell epitheliomas having been present for 10 years or longer with little evidence of growth. Likewise, sebaceous cell carcinomas may mimic chalazia.

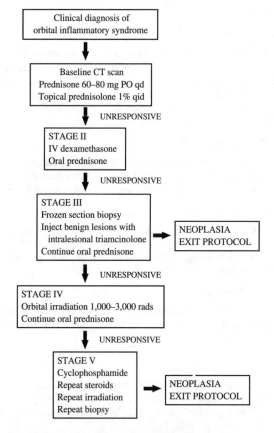

Fig. 4.1 Flow diagram for treatment of orbital inflammatory syndrome. (Modified from CR Leone Jr, WC Lloyd. Treatment protocol for inflammatory disease. Ophthalmology 1985;92:1325–1331.)

Malignant Tumors

Basal Cell Epithelioma

Basal cell epithelioma is the most common eyelid tumor. It tends to appear on the lower lid or medial canthus. Most are nodular with a characteristic pearly surface and telangiectatic vessels. This tumor may show central ulceration and may also present in morphea or sclerosing form that typically appears flat and leathery and is particularly infiltrative. Metastatic spread is rare.

Squamous Cell Carcinoma

Squamous cell carcinomas have variable appearances; they can be nodular or ulcerated, usually with distinct borders. They often arise from actinic keratosis and occasionally metastasize to regional lymph nodes.

Sebaceous Cell Carcinoma

Sebaceous cell carcinoma arises most often from the meibomian glands. Its growth may mimic chalazia or may be multifocal. Orbital extension and metastasis are not uncommon. A referral to an internist for metastatic workup is recommended.

Malignant Melanoma

Malignant melanoma is uncommon on the eyelid. It may arise from preexisting nevi; it commonly metastasizes; and it may have irregular borders and color.

Key Points

- Malignant tumors tend to destroy normal lid architecture and accessory appendages (e.g., lashes, meibomian glands).
- A Moh's micrographic surgery may be useful for recurrent or morpheaform basal cell epitheliomas.
- The skip areas seen with sebaceous adenocarcinoma make map biopsies more useful for this neoplasm.
- Regional lymph node dissection may be necessary for cutaneous melanomas that show microscopic evidence of vascular or lym-

phatic involvement. Melanomas greater than 1.5 mm in thickness mandate a metastatic workup and oncology consultation.

- When the diagnosis is in doubt, it may be wise to perform an incisional biopsy to possibly avoid cosmetic or functional problems associated with wide surgical excision.
- Excised lid lesions should be sent for histologic examination. The margins of histologically malignant lesions need to be examined to see that the tumor was not transected.
- Be suspicious of sebaceous cell carcinoma in cases of recurrent chalazia.

Benign Eyelid Tumors

Cysts

Cysts may be epidermal inclusions or sudoriferous or sebaceous in nature. The cysts' margins are well circumscribed and may be surgically excised.

Keratoacanthoma

Keratoacanthoma is a benign tumor characterized by very rapid growth and may be confused with basal cell epithelioma. Typically, it is nodular with a central ulcer crater. Often it shrinks and resolves spontaneously, but surgical excision is warranted when the lid margin is involved because of the potential for tissue destruction.

Molluscum Contagiosum

Molluscum contagiosum is sometimes confused with basal cell epithelioma. It appears as papules with an umbilicated center from which a cheesy material may be expressed. It is the result of infection by pox virus and may produce a keratoconjunctivitis. Treatment is curettage or surgical excision.

Verrucae

A verruca is a common papillary tumor often with a cauliflower-like appearance to its surface. It is caused by the papovavirus and may cause a keratoconjunctivitis when the lid margin is involved. Treatment is surgical excision or chemical destruction with bichloracetic acid (not with lid margin lesions).

Nevus

A nevus is a flat or elevated, often pigmented tumor containing nevus cells. It is well circumscribed and sometimes has hair. A careful history and documentation on follow-up are necessary to rule out growth and malignant transformation.

Seborrheic Keratosis

Seborrheic keratosis is usually a brown-black, greasy-scaly–appearing lesion with a "stuck-on" appearance and is seen in older individuals. It may be removed with a shave biopsy. This tumor should be differentiated from actinic keratosis, which tends to have ill-defined borders and is considered a premalignant cancer that may transform into squamous cell carcinoma.

EYELID MYOKYMIA

Myokymia is a unilateral twitching of the lid, often more noticeable to the patient than the examiner. Myokymia may be precipitated by fatigue, anemia, or ocular irritation. Reassurance, proper rest, and stable caffeine intake are often adequate treatment for myokymia. Promethazine 12.5–25.0 mg 1–3 times a day, or tripelennamine 75 mg 4 times a day may be tried for recalcitrant or severe cases of myokymia.

BENIGN ESSENTIAL BLEPHAROSPASM

Blepharospasm is a bilateral, uncontrolled blinking or closure of the eyelids. It occurs most commonly in women over the age of 50.

Signs and Symptoms

Benign essential blepharospasm consists of bilateral involuntary contractures of the orbicularis oculi that vary in intensity from small twitches to forceful contractures. The contractures disappear during sleep.

Management

- Differentiate from other conditions of lid twitch or closure (see Chap. 1).
- Botulinum toxin injections are effective for many patients with benign essential blepharospasm but need to be repeated every 3–6 months.

HEMIFACIAL SPASM

Unlike blepharospasm, hemifacial spasm is usually a unilateral condition. It is characterized by synchronous contractions of the entire side of the face. In most cases, the etiology is vascular compression of the facial nerve at the brain stem.

Signs and Symptoms

- Intermittent unilateral facial contractions that persist during sleep
- Like blepharospasm, it is more common in middle-aged women.
- There is often an associated facial nerve weakness.

Management

- Magnetic resonance imaging and magnetic resonance angiography should be performed to rule out pontine glioma or identify an ectatic vessel.
- Neurosurgical decompression of the facial nerve can be curative in some cases.
- Botulinum toxin injections may be useful for those cases in which surgery is not an option.

THYROID EYE DISEASE

Grave's ophthalmopathy is an autoimmune disease characterized by the production of antibodies that stimulate the thyroid gland. It should be kept in mind that many of the ophthalmic manifestations of Graves' disease (e.g., proptosis, ocular motility disturbances from involvement of the extraocular muscles) are a result of the underlying autoimmune disease rather than a result of hyperthyroidism. Therefore, it is possible to display the signs and symptoms of Graves' disease even though the patient is euthyroid or even hypothyroid. Also, while ablation of the thyroid gland may correct hyperthyroidism, the patient with Graves' disease may show progression of ophthalmopathy.

Differential Diagnosis

CT scanning of the orbit can be helpful in differentiating thyroid eye disease from other causes of proptosis. OIS (myositis) is characterized by diffuse enlargement of the extraocular muscles. Characteristically the tendons are spared in thyroid-related orbitopathy. Thyroid function may be evaluated by measuring the serum thyroid-stimulating hormone and the free thyroxine index. Thyroid immune evaluation is via thyroid-stimulating immunoglobulin and antithyroid antibodies (e.g., antithyroglobulin, antithyroid peroxidase).

Treatment

- Treat exposure keratopathy with artificial tears 4–12 times a day (see the section on management of dry eyes).
- Severe proptosis, restriction of extraocular muscles, and resultant diplopia may necessitate oral steroids or muscle surgery.
- Optic neuropathy is an urgent situation. Systemic steroids, radiation therapy, and/or posterior orbital decompression all may be part of the management.

HISTIOCYTOSIS X

Histiocytosis X represents a spectrum of disorders, ranging from benign lesions to potentially fatal dissemination. It is characterized by proliferating histiocytes (macrophages) and is found most often in children. Other names for this disorder include Langerhans' cell histiocytosis, eosinophilic granuloma, Hand-Schüller-Christian, and Letterer-Siwe disease (depending on malignant potential and dissemination). When the orbit is involved, it can lead to proptosis and soft-tissue swelling and inflammation.

Signs and Symptoms

- Proptosis
- Soft-tissue swelling
- Lytic lesion on CT scanning

Management

- Workup for systemic involvement (more common for children presenting under age 2)
- Confirmational biopsy
- Debulking
- Intralesional steroid injection or low-dose radiation
- Regular monitoring to rule out multiorgan involvement
- Bones usually completely reossify after treatment.

CAPILLARY HEMANGIOMAS

Capillary hemangiomas are common benign vascular tumors of the orbit that affect young children. They have a predilection for the superonasal quadrant of the orbit and upper eyelid. Capillary hemangiomas of the lid or orbit may cause amblyopia by occlusion, production of strabismus, or induction of astigmatism. The Kassabach-Merritt syndrome refers to thrombocytopenia in association with large hemangiomas. Capillary hemangiomas become manifest during the first year of life. They are often the source of much parental consternation, but 75% of these lesions involute by the time the patient is age 5.

Signs and Symptoms

- Superficial tumors produce strawberry discoloration of the skin.
- Deeper lesions produce bluish discoloration.
- They often produce ptosis.

- CT scanning cannot always distinguish from other tumors such as rhabdomyosarcoma.

Management

- Monitor visual acuity and refractive error.
- Amblyopia therapy as needed
- When therapy is necessary:
  1. Local (often repeat) steroid injections (betamethasone and triamcinolone). Potential side effects include skin necrosis, fat atrophy, growth retardation, and vision loss from emboli.
  2. Systemic steroids
  3. Surgical excision
  4. Systemic alpha-interferon
  5. Radiation therapy. Potential side effects include cataract formation, depressed bone growth, and production of malignancies.

RHABDOMYOSARCOMA

Rhabdomyosarcoma is the most common primary orbital malignancy in children. It is often mistaken for more benign conditions such as preseptal cellulitis, capillary hemangiomas, and swelling due to coincidental trauma.

Signs and Symptoms

- Often sudden, unilateral proptosis but may follow more gradual course (weeks)
- Often associated edema and discoloration of lids
- May be a palpable mass
- Often with bone destruction on CT scanning
- Most commonly affects retrobulbar or superonasal quadrant
- Average age of patient is 7–8 years.

Types (Based on Microscopic Examination)

- Embryonal is the most common form.

- Alveolar is the most malignant form and has a predilection for the inferior orbit.
- Pleomorphic is the rarest form and occurs in older patients. This type has the best prognosis.
- Botryoid is a rare variant of the embryonal type with a grapelike form. It is a secondary invader of the orbit from the paranasal sinuses or conjunctiva.

Management

- CT scan of the orbits
- Immediate biopsy
- Rule out metastases with palpation of cervical and preauricular lymph nodes, chest x-ray, bone marrow aspirate and biopsy, and lumbar puncture.
- Surgical debulking of the tumor may be helpful, but the mainstay of treatment is radiation therapy and systemic chemotherapy.

NOTES

5

The Cornea

CORNEAL DYSTROPHIES

Corneal dystrophies are bilateral hereditary disorders not associated with systemic disease. Table 5.1 can be used as a guide in making a differential diagnosis. Examining other family members may be helpful in making the correct diagnosis, especially in early disease.

Treatment

1. For ocular discomfort, foreign body sensation, recurrent erosions:
   - Ocular lubricants—e.g., artificial tears, bland ophthalmic ointments
   - Hypertonic sodium chloride drops and ointment
   - Soft contact lenses can sometimes be beneficial
   - Stromal puncture for recalcitrant cases of recurrent erosion
2. For decreased visual acuity:
   - Hypertonic sodium chloride for corneal edema
   - A reduction of intraocular pressure can be helpful in Fuchs' dystrophy.
   - Gently blow hair dryer toward eyes for 5–10 minutes in the morning to dehydrate the cornea.
   - Lamellar keratoplasty or superficial keratectomy for superficial opacities
   - Penetrating keratoplasty for deeper opacities

KERATOCONUS

Keratoconus is characterized by conical bulging (ectasia) of the central cornea. With progression, it becomes thinned and scarred and is

Table 5.1   Corneal Dystrophies

Dystrophy	Level	Inheritance	Clinical Features
Meesman's	Epithelium	AD	Tiny gray-white punctuate opacities/cysts in intrapalpebral zone; minimal symptoms and acuity loss
Cogan's microcytic (map, dot, fingerprint)	Epithelial BM	AD, variable penetrance	Intraepithelial lines, dots, maps; minimal blur, foreign body sensation, recurrent erosion
Reis-Buckler's	Bowman's	AD	Epithelial alterations over interwoven ring opacities; recurrent erosions; decreased VA in 20s age group
Crystalline	Stroma	AD	Early onset; fine-needle–shaped, colored crystals; minimal effect on VA; no discomfort
Granular	Stroma	AD	Irregular white opacities appear in first decade of life; VA drops as intervening stroma clouds (30s to 40s)
Macular	Stroma	AR	Multiple gray-white opacities at all levels of the stroma; severe vision loss by fifth decade of life. May show recurrent erosions and irregular astigmatism
Lattice	Stroma	AD	Refractile anterior stromal branching lines, dots with sparing of periphery; ocular lubricants
Fuchs'	Endothelium/epithelium	AD	More common in females; corneal guttata in third to sixth decade of life, possibly progressing to corneal edema and bullae
Posterior polymorphous	Endothelium	AD or AR	Grouped vesicles at Descemet's membrane; often asymmetric; irregular white patches; minimal effect on acuity

AD = autosomal dominant; BM = basement membrane; AR = autosomal recessive; VA = visual acuity.

associated with irregular astigmatism. There is no definite inheritance pattern.

Clinical Signs

- Progressive steepening/astigmatism of the cornea; often irregular
- Distortion of retinoscopic reflex/keratometric mires
- Increased visibility of corneal stromal nerves

 With progression, the patient may have:

- Vertical corneal striae
- Axial thinning
- Fleisher ring (iron)
- Munson's sign (bulging of lower lid in downgaze)
- Corneal hydrops (sudden corneal edema from Descemet's rupture)

Treatment

- Correct refractive error with spectacles or rigid gas-permeable contact lenses.
- For corneal hydrops: 1% or 2% cyclopentolate (cycloplegia), 5% sodium chloride ointment and pressure patch. Follow with hypertonic sodium chloride for several days until edema clears.
- Corneal surgery for severe scarring and poor vision with contact lens intolerance

MARGINAL DEGENERATIONS AND ULCERS

A variety of disorders may directly affect the peripheral cornea. Differentiation from peripheral corneal disorders secondary to systemic conditions is important for both prognosis and management.

Terrien's Marginal Degeneration

- Typically a bilateral condition characterized by nonulcerative thinning of the peripheral cornea

- Opacification, thinning, and vascularization of the involved corneal segment
- Lipid deposits may be seen at the leading edge and usually involve the superior cornea.
- May lead to progressive astigmatism, which can be corrected with eyeglasses or contact lenses
- Spontaneous perforation is rare; typically only with mild irritation that can be treated with topical lubricants.

Furrow Degeneration

- Furrow degeneration is a benign condition seen in older patients. It presents as a peripheral corneal thinning seen in the area of an arcus senilis.
- There is no ulceration, inflammation, or vascularization.
- Topical lubricants can be prescribed for any resulting irritation.

Pellucid Marginal Degeneration

- Bilateral, clear corneal thinning associated
- Inferior cornea most commonly involved
- Most commonly diagnosed in patients 20 years to 40 years of age
- May develop high irregular astigmatism as in keratoconus
- Acute hydrops may develop.
- Unlike keratoconus, corneal protrusion is above the area of maximal thinning.
- Treatment with contact lenses, penetrating keratoplasty, and so forth is similar to that for keratoconus.

Mooren's Ulcer

- An idiopathic, painful, ulcerating, peripheral corneal condition with inflammation that tends to run a progressive course
- Typically, there is an overhanging edge of an epithelial defect with vascularization of the ulcer base.
- Advancement of the ulceration is both peripheral around the limbus and central.

- A particularly aggressive form of Mooren's ulcer is seen in young Nigerian black males. It is more commonly bilateral and often associated with parasitemia.
- Diagnosis can only be made after other systemic diseases associated with peripheral ulceration have been ruled out (see the section on corneal thinning from collagen vascular disease below).
- Treatment may include topical steroids, systemic steroids, immunosuppressive agents, and conjunctival excision and recession with or without cryotherapy of the recessed edge.
- Topical antibiotic drops may be used prophylactically to prevent infection.
- Perforation can occur. Corneal grafts have a tendency to melt or vascularize. Cyanoacrylate adhesive or surgery, or both, may be necessary in perforation or impending perforation.

Corneal Thinning from Collagen Vascular Disease

- Rheumatoid arthritis, systemic lupus erythematosus, Wegener's granulomatosis, polyarteritis nodosa, and relapsing polychondritis may all be associated with a peripheral ulcerative keratitis.
- Workup may include a complete blood count, erythrocyte sedimentation rate, C-reactive protein, antinuclear antibody, anti–double-stranded DNA, rheumatoid factor, antineutrophil cytoplasmic antibodies, and chest x-ray.
- Typically, there is an epithelial defect with inflammatory thinning of the peripheral cornea.
- The ulcers may progress circumferentially and perforation may occur.
- In general, use of topical steroids is discouraged because they may lead to progressive melting and perforation.
- Treatment involves ocular lubricants, cycloplegics, and systemic steroids.
- Immunosuppressive agents may be useful, especially in Wegener's granulomatosis.
- Excision of adjacent conjunctiva may be beneficial.
- For corneal perforation or impending perforation, consider cyanoacrylate adhesive, corneal transplant, or conjunctival flaps.

CALCIFIC BAND KERATOPATHY

Calcific band keratopathy is a degeneration of the superficial cornea that results in deposition of calcium hydroxyapatite, mainly in Bowman's layer. It appears as a horizontal band of white calcium, usually appearing first in the peripheral cornea. Usually there is a peripheral clear zone between the limbus and the peripheral edge of the keratopathy.

Etiology

- Chronic uveitis or other chronic inflammatory eye disease
- Hypercalcemia
- Hereditary
- Elevated serum phosphorus (e.g., as in renal disease)
- Chronic use of ophthalmic medications with mercury preservatives
- Silicone oil use in an aphakic eye

Management

- Treatment of any underlying condition
- Early in its course, lubrication with artificial tears and ointment may keep the eye more comfortable and maintain vision.
- More advanced cases may require chelation. This is performed by applying disodium ethylenediaminetetraacetic acid to Bowman's layer after the epithelium has been removed. Removal may be aided by mechanical scraping. The proper concentration of ethylenediaminetetraacetic acid (EDTA) may be obtained by mixing one 5-ml vial of EDTA, 150 mg per ml, with 100 ml of sterile ophthalmic irrigation solution.
- The use of the excimer laser for removal has also been described.

PHLYCTENULOSIS

Phlyctenulosis is an inflammatory condition of the paralimbal tissue believed to be a hypersensitivity response to an antigen, historically to tuberculosis but in the United States most commonly to *Staphylococcus aureus.* Most commonly it affects children and young adults.

Signs and Symptoms

- Nodular pink or white gelatinous lesion of the conjunctiva or cornea often in the interpalpebral area
- Corneal phlyctenules often present with a leash of vessels leading to it from the limbus
- There may be necrosis of the center of the lesion, and the lesion may migrate across the cornea.
- There may be complaints of itching, burning, and photophobia.
- There may be signs of an associated bacterial keratoconjunctivitis.
- Multiple, chronic, or recurrent phlyctenules can result in corneal scarring and permanent vision loss, but the lesion usually remains superficial. Perforation is rare.

Management

- Search for associated conditions such as tuberculosis and perform a workup in high-risk patients. Consider chlamydia. Ask about a history of herpes simplex keratitis. Look for evidence of acne rosacea or staphylococcal blepharokeratoconjunctivitis. Phlyctenulosis is rarely associated with intestinal parasites or coccidioidomycosis.
- In addition to treatment of the associated condition, resolution of the lesion and limitation of scarring can be accomplished with the use of topical steroids (e.g., fluorometholone 0.1% [FML] qid with a slow taper). This may not be appropriate in association with herpes simplex.
- Treat empirically with a topical antistaphylococcal antibiotic. Bacitracin ointment 2–3 times a day may be a good choice. Oral tetracycline or erythromycin is appropriate for chlamydia, ocular rosacea, or chronic staphylococcal infection. These oral agents can produce long-term remission in difficult cases, even when the associated disorder is in doubt. Using tetracycline, 250 mg tid for 3 weeks, then once a day for 2 months, is one method to obtain remission.

- Erythromycin 25 mg/kg in 4 divided dosages should be substituted for the above in children younger than 8 years of age.

EPITHELIAL KERATITIS

Epithelial keratitis is not a diagnosis but a descriptive term for superficial corneal inflammation. Epithelial keratitis is usually, but not invariably, associated with fluorescein staining. The distribution and pattern of epithelial involvement can be of tremendous value in determining the underlying etiology (Fig. 5.1).

RECURRENT CORNEAL EROSIONS

Recurrent corneal erosions are characterized by spontaneous sloughing of the corneal epithelium. Often there is a remote history of injury with a sharp object. Many patients have epithelial basement membrane dystrophy.

Signs and Symptoms

- Patients may present with the acute onset of pain, often upon awakening.
- There is often evidence of a healing epithelial erosion.
- Aberrant epithelial regeneration may manifest as irregular epithelium, mounds, or strands of epithelium (filaments), or microcysts and bullae.

Treatment

- Acute episodes can be managed by patching with antibiotic ointment until there is healing of the epithelial defect. Long-term,

Fig. 5.1 ▶ Epithelial keratitis. The pattern of keratitis can provide important clues regarding the underlying etiology. (Reprinted with permission from D Vaughan. General Ophthalmology [13th ed.]. Norwalk, CT: Appleton & Lange, 1993.)

Minute fluorescein-staining erosions; lower third of cornea affected predominantly. 1. Staphylococcal keratitis	Typically dendritic (occasionally round or oval) with edema and degeneration. 2. Herpetic keratitis (HSK)	More diffuse than lesions of HSK; occasionally linear (pseudodendrites). 3. Varicella-zoster keratitis
Minute fluorescein-staining erosions; diffuse but most conspicuous in pupillary area. 4. Adenovirus keratitis	Minute pleomorphic, fluorescein-staining, damaged epithelium and erosions; epithelial and mucous filaments are typical; lower half of cornea affected predominantly. 5. Keratitis of Sjögren's syndrome	Minute fluorescein-staining, irregular erosions; lower half of cornea affected predominantly. 6. Exposure keratitis—due to lagophthalmos or exophthalmos
Blotchy gray, opaque, syncytiumlike lesions, most conspicuous in upper pupillary area. Sometimes a plaque of opaque epithelium forms. 7. Vernal keratoconjunctivitis	Blotchy epithelial edema; diffuse but predominant in palpebral fissure, 9–3 o'clock. 8. Trophic keratitis—sequela of herpes simplex, herpes zoster, and gasserian ganglion destruction	Minute fluorescein-staining erosions with spotty cellular edema; highly characteristic picture. 9. Drug-induced keratitis—especially by broad-spectrum antibiotics
Foci of edematous epithelial cells, round or oval; elevated when disease is active. 10. Superficial punctate keratitis (SPK)	Minute fluorescein-staining erosions of upper third of cornea; filaments during exacerbations; bulbar hyperemia, thickened limbus, micropannus. 11. Superior limbic keratoconjunctivitis	Virus-type lesions like those of SPK; in pupillary area. 12. Rubeola, rubella, and mumps keratitis
Minute fluorescein-staining epithelial erosions affecting upper third of cornea. 13. Trachoma		Spotty gray opacification of individual epithelial cells due to partial keratinization; associated with Bitot's spots. 14. Vitamin A deficiency keratitis

nightly applications of bland ophthalmic ointment are sometimes successful in preventing recurrent episodes.
- Application of 5% sodium chloride ophthalmic ointment on a daily basis is thought by some authorities to be helpful.
- An extended-wear contact lens can be used when more conservative methods fail to bring relief.
- Resistant cases can be treated with anterior stromal puncture with a needle or YAG laser. Phototherapeutic keratectomy with the excimer laser is another option.

FILAMENTARY KERATOPATHY

Filamentary keratopathy is characterized by strands of mucus and degenerating epithelial cells attached to the cornea. The condition is associated with dry eye and other chronic ocular surface conditions. The condition is also often seen in comatose patients and in neurotrophic keratopathy.

Signs and Symptoms

- Pain and foreign body sensation
- Epithelial and mucus strands, often more concentrated on the superior cornea

Treatment

- Debridement with forceps after the application of topical anesthetic. Five percent sodium chloride ophthalmic ointment applied daily is thought by some authorities to be helpful.
- Lubrication with nonpreserved artificial tears or bland ophthalmic ointment
- Resistant cases can be treated with a bandage contact lens, although this is not recommended in cases of neurotrophic keratopathy.

CORNEAL DELLEN

Dellens are localized areas of corneal thinning often associated with ocular surface abnormalities. They are commonly seen after ocular surgery (e.g., pterygium excision). They are a result of local drying.

Signs and Symptoms

- Patients may complain of a foreign body sensation or pain. Conjunctival injection is common.
- The dellen appears as an oval area of corneal excavation near the limbus with fluorescein pooling or staining.
- There is often an adjacent region of conjunctival irregularity or elevation.

Treatment

- Lubrication with bland ophthalmic ointment or patching with antibiotic ointment until there is resolution. Long-term lubrication with artificial tears or ointment may be necessary to prevent recurrence.
- On occasion, surgical revision of the conjunctival irregularity or a lateral tarsorrhaphy may be necessary.

THYGESON'S SUPERFICIAL PUNCTATE KERATOPATHY

Thygeson's superficial punctate keratopathy is a disease of uncertain etiology characterized by recurrent episodes of keratopathy not associated with concurrent or past conjunctivitis.

Signs

- Punctate, white epithelial opacities, slightly elevated with negative staining on the central cornea

- Minimal or no conjunctival injection
- Foreign body sensation
- Often bilateral

Treatment

- Artificial tears 4–6 times a day and bland ophthalmic ointment (e.g., Lacri-Lube) at bedtime
- Mild topical steroid (e.g., fluorometholone 0.1% or 0.125% prednisolone 4 times a day)

SUPERIOR LIMBIC KERATOCONJUNCTIVITIS

Superior limbic keratoconjunctivitis is associated with contact lens wear or is idiopathic in nature.

Clinical Signs

- Conjunctival and/or corneal staining with fluorescein/rose bengal in the region of the superior limbus
- Conjunctival injection
- Papillae of superior tarsal conjunctiva
- May show superior micropannus or corneal filaments
- Foreign body sensation
- Often bilateral, chronic, and recurrent

Management

- Fifty percent of patients with non–contact lens–associated superior limbic keratoconjunctivitis have dysthyroid disease, so thyroid function studies (triiodothyronine, thyroxine, and thyroid-stimulating hormone) should be performed.
- Administer artificial tears 4–6 times a day with bland ophthalmic ointment (e.g., Lacri-Lube) at bedtime for mild cases.
- Try therapeutic soft contact lens for non–contact lens–associated disease.
- For more severe cases, try silver nitrate in a 0.5–1.0% solution (from wax ampules) applied to the superior tarsus and conjunctiva with a

cotton-tipped applicator (anesthetize with proparacaine before treatment).
- Cryotherapy, cautery, or surgical resection may be necessary for severe, otherwise unresponsive cases.

BULLOUS KERATOPATHY

Bullous keratopathy is often a form of corneal decompensation seen after intraocular surgery. It may result from ocular inflammation or trauma to the corneal endothelium, or it may be seen in patients with preexisting Fuchs' dystrophy.

Clinical Signs

- Corneal edema, striae, and clouding
- Corneal bullae possibly with endothelial guttata
- Possible episodes of sharp pain from rupture of bullae

Management

- Reduce intraocular pressure if elevated (topical beta blocker such as timolol or betaxolol bid). Avoid epinephrine as it may precipitate cystoid macular edema.
- Five percent sodium chloride drops 4–6 times a day with ointment at bedtime.
- Ruptured bullae may be treated as corneal abrasion (see Chap. 2).
- In nonresponsive cases in which corneal surgery must be deferred, a bandage contact lens may be used to manage bullae and erosions resulting from their rupture.
- Corneal transplant surgery for patients with poor vision or pain and no signs of recovery.

ACANTHAMOEBA

Acanthamoeba is a free-living protozoan that can cause keratitis or sclerokeratitis after corneal injury and contact with contaminated water or contact lens solutions.

Risk Factors

- Contact lens wearers, especially those using distilled water, homemade saline, tap water, or well water or who wet their contacts with saliva
- Corneal injuries associated with a contaminated foreign body or with submersion in hot tubs, lakes, or other fresh-water sources

Signs and Symptoms

- Most often misdiagnosed as herpes simplex keratitis
- Early on may show pseudodendritic keratitis; branching superficial corneal opacities
- Often show inflammatory "cuffing" of corneal nerves (radial keratoneuritis)
- May progress to patchy stromal infiltrates, disciform keratitis and characteristic stromal ring infiltrate; corneal perforation is common
- Anterior uveitis or nodular scleritis, or both, may also present.

Laboratory Diagnosis

- Culture of solutions and corneal scrapings on non-nutrient agar plates precoated with *Escherichia coli.*
- Scrapings and/or tissue biopsy with calcofluor white or immunofluorescent antibody staining.
- Various other stains may also identify the organism or cysts including Gram's, Giemsa, hematoxylin-eosin, and Wright's.

Management

- Treatment is difficult. There is no established, well-accepted treatment regimen.
- 0.1% Propamidine (Brolene) (available in Great Britain but investigational in the United States) 1 drop every hour, *plus*
- Neomycin, polymyxin B, and gramicidin ophthalmic solution 1 drop every hour, *plus*

- Polyhexamethylene biguanide (Baquacil), a swimming pool cleaner, 1:1,000 in artificial tears 1 drop every hour
- The above triple regimen should be continued for 1–3 days and may gradually be tapered to every 4 hours over the next 1–3 weeks.
- Brolene and Baquacil should be continued once a day for 6–12 months.
- 1% Clotrimazole suspension, formulated from a powder in artificial tears, has also been described in the successful management of *Acanthamoeba.*
- Penetrating keratoplasty is often necessary, even after successful management.

HERPES SIMPLEX KERATITIS

In clinical practice, the practitioner is much more likely to encounter recurrent herpes simplex keratitis than primary infection. The latter occurs most frequently in young children and may show little in the way of signs or symptoms. Reactivation of latent virus may be precipitated by illness or immunosuppressive agents and manifests itself as epithelial or stromal disease.

Epithelial Disease

Epithelial keratitis may begin as small opaque areas on the epithelial surface. Coalescence of the localized keratitis may result in linear, stellate, or dendritic patterns. Terminal end bulbs, slightly elevated ulcer margins that stain with rose bengal, and relative corneal hypoesthesia are helpful in differentiating epithelial disease from other disorders. Geographic keratitis appears most commonly in immunocompromised individuals or as a result of steroid therapy.

Stromal Keratitis

Stromal keratitis may be the result of an immunologic reaction to a viral antigen that has found its way into the corneal stroma. It may manifest itself as an interstitial keratitis with limbal infiltrates and vascularization. Alternatively, it may appear as a localized area of corneal edema, sometimes accompanied by deep folds, bullae, and/or keratic precipitates. This so-called disciform keratitis may be accompanied by a concurrent iridocyclitis or trabeculitis with secondary inflammatory glaucoma or necrotic stromal thinning, or both.

Laboratory Studies

- Rarely indicated
- Viral cultures (media should be kept on ice)
- Immunofluorescent assay

Because 90% of the U.S. population has been infected with the herpes virus, there is no reliable method to substantiate stromal herpes. A negative serology would mitigate against herpes as the etiologic agent in a stromal keratitis.

Therapy

Epithelial

- Minimal wipe debridement (roll cotton-tipped applicator over dendrite)
- Topical antiviral agents; trifluridine 1 drop 8 or 9 times a day appears to be the most effective. Continue until dendrites disappear. Taper to qid for 4–7 days.
- Cycloplegics for comfort or mild secondary iritis if indicated.

Stromal

Stromal keratitis should only be handled by clinicians with considerable experience. It may be desirable to manage stromal keratitis without topical steroids, because patients tend to become steroid-dependent. For first episodes and stromal involvement outside visual axis try:

- Trifluridine 1 drop every 2 hours

If, after 1 week, stromal involvement affects the visual axis, try:

- Trifluridine and prednisolone 0.125% on 1:1 basis

For nonresponsive cases or patients with known steroid dependence or concurrent significant uveitis:

- Steroid with antiviral agent on a 1:1 basis depending on severity

Depending on circumstances:

- Cycloplegics
- Beta blocker or carbonic anhydrase inhibitor if there is a secondary rise in intraocular pressure
- Very slow tapering of steroids

HERPES ZOSTER OPHTHALMICUS

Herpes zoster, or shingles, is a well-known cause of keratoconjunctivitis, iritis, scleritis, and trabeculitis. It is caused by the varicella zoster (chickenpox) virus. The etiology of the ocular condition is seldom in question because it is almost always accompanied by the characteristic unilateral skin vesicles, which respect the facial midline.

In addition to oral acyclovir and possibly oral steroids and analgesic agents for cutaneous involvement, ocular involvement may require specific therapy.

Conjunctivitis

Usually only supportive therapy is indicated for inflammation localized to the conjunctiva. Topical astringents and lubricants can be beneficial. Mild steroids such as prednisolone 0.125% may be indicated for patient comfort.

Keratitis

Epithelial dendritic and stellate lesions that mimic those of simplex keratitis may be present. The cornea can also demonstrate raised white mucous plaques or stromal edema. The treatment in all cases is the application of topical corticosteroids in proportion to the severity of inflammation. Epithelial keratitis may respond to prednisolone 0.125% 3–4 times a day, whereas stromal keratitis may require prednisolone 1% as often as hourly. Topical antibiotics may be used if a secondary bacterial infection is suspected. Corneal melting and thinning may call for more aggressive therapy such as contact lenses or cyanoacrylate glue.

Iritis and Scleritis

Topical steroids are the mainstay of treatment for iritis and scleritis. Occasionally oral anti-inflammatory drugs may be needed. Uveitis and scleritis may require treatment for months.

Glaucoma

A secondary glaucoma is not uncommonly associated with keratitis or uveitis. Most often the cause is an associated trabeculitis. Treatment is topical steroids in association with topical beta blockers or oral antiglaucoma medications, or both. The clinician also needs to be aware of the possibility of steroid response from prolonged administration of these medications.

Other Disorders

In addition to the disorders discussed above, choroiditis, optic neuritis, and cranial nerve palsy are also possibilities. Ocular examinations should rule out these other less common associated disorders.

CORNEAL GRAFT REJECTION

Prompt, aggressive treatment of graft rejection episodes provides the greatest likelihood of graft survival. Rejection of corneal grafts after penetrating keratoplasty takes one of three forms:

1. Endothelial rejection. Signs and symptoms are:
   - Inflammatory precipitates on the endothelium (scattered, fine, random clumps, or linear [Khodadoust line])
   - Decreased vision, photophobia

- Conjunctival erythema
- Corneal thickening, edema, clouding
- Epithelial edema
2. Subepithelial infiltrates, which may be asymptomatic and can be associated with an anterior chamber reaction
3. Epithelial rejection, with which an elevated epithelial ridge develops

Management

- Frequent topical steroid administration (e.g., prednisolone 1% up to 1 drop every 15 minutes, depending on severity)
- Cyclosporine 1–2% has also been used both for prophylaxis and treatment of graft rejection.

CORNEAL ULCER

Numerous authorities have offered advice on differentiating infectious from noninfectious (sterile) corneal ulceration.

Sterile corneal ulcers are generally an immune response to bacterial toxins or other antigens or a response to hypoxia, as in contact lens wearers. They are usually found in the peripheral cornea and are separated from the limbus by a small zone of clear cornea. Sterile infiltrates are more likely to be free of stain and may show less surrounding edema.

Infectious ulcers tend to be characterized by more pain and are more likely to show an anterior chamber reaction. If there is any doubt, the ulcer should be treated as infectious.

Bacterial Corneal Ulcer

Suspected bacterial corneal ulcers should be cultured at the first visit to eliminate the possibility that antibiotic use will interfere with laboratory studies.

Recommended Culture Technique

1. Use a sterile, moistened cotton-tipped applicator and wipe along the lower cul-de-sac (use sterile saline from an aerosol can or trypticase-

soy broth to wet the applicator). Inoculate a sheep blood and chocolate agar plate, making a row of small letter c's on each agar plate.
2. After instilling a topical anesthetic agent, the ulcer itself should
   be scraped using a dry calcium alginate or Dacron-tipped applicator. Make another row of c's on the sheep blood and chocolate
   agar plates. After making another pass over the ulcer, break the
   applicator tip into a tube of thioglycolate medium.
3. Sterilize (flame) a platinum spatula and scrape the ulcer again.
   Smear the specimen onto at least two microscopic slides for
   Gram's and Giemsa or other special stains.
4. After another pass with the spatula, inoculate the sheep blood,
   chocolate, and Sabouraud's agar plates.
5. Other media (such as Löwenstein-Jensen for mycobacterium)
   can be used if there is any reason to suspect more unusual
   organisms.

Therapy

Most corneal ulcers can effectively be managed on an outpatient
basis, assuming perforation is not imminent and patient compliance
can reasonably be assured.

Whereas some authorities choose to base initial therapeutic decisions on preliminary Gram stain results, another method is to use
both fortified tobramycin and vancomycin or cefazolin eyedrops in
cases of suspected bacterial keratitis in an effort to achieve a broad
spectrum of coverage. Alternating the drops every 30 minutes during
waking hours and then applying one drop of each every 2 hours at
night is a method to obtain high drug concentration.

Ciprofloxin and ofloxacin are commercially available topical
antibiotics that can be effective in the treatment of corneal ulcers
caused by susceptible organisms (see the ophthalmic pharmaceutical
tables in Chap. 22).

The use of a collagen shield or hydrophilic contact lens can act to
further increase drug concentration and contact time. It is questionable
whether subconjunctival administration of these drugs provides any

additional advantage over topical administration alone. Therapy can be altered once laboratory results and/or clinical improvement is noted.

The clinician should always be aware of the toxicity of the drugs and not mistake the almost inevitable ocular inflammation that results from the drugs for worsening of the infectious keratitis. Instructions for preparing these medications for topical application are provided below.

Fortified Drug Preparation

Cefazolin
Add 5 ml sterile normal saline to a 1-g vial of cefazolin sodium powder for injection. Swirl (do not shake) into solution. With syringe, withdraw solution and inject into 15-ml dropper bottle of artificial tears. Rapid degradation requires that new cefazolin drops be prepared every 2–3 days.

Tobramycin
Withdraw contents of a 2-ml vial of tobramycin sulfate (40 mg/ml) injection with a syringe and inject into 5-ml dropper bottle of 0.3% tobramycin, resulting in a final concentration of approximately 14 mg/ml.

Vancomycin
Withdraw 2 ml of artificial tears from a 15-ml bottle and inject into a 500-mg vial of vancomycin. Withdraw this reconstituted vancomycin and inject it into the bottle of artificial tears.

Amphotericin B
Usual concentration is 0.5–5.0 mg/ml. Dilute parenteral drug with distilled water.

NOTES

6

Uveitis

ENDOPHTHALMITIS (POST–CATARACT SURGERY)

One of the most dreaded complications of cataract surgery is infectious endophthalmitis. The presentation varies depending on the etiologic agent.

Sterile endophthalmitis refers to an inflammatory response to retained crystalline lens material, chemicals, or foreign bodies introduced at the time of surgery or the intraocular lens material. The inflammation is generally not as severe as that seen in infectious endophthalmitis.

Infectious endophthalmitis generally appears as an increasing inflammatory response during the first week after surgery. Exceptions include infections with *Propionibacterium acnes* and fungal organisms that may present later and follow a more indolent course.

SIGNS AND SYMPTOMS

Not all signs or symptoms need be present.

- Decreased vision
- Pain
- Anterior chamber reaction, sometimes with hypopyon
- Vitreitis
- Lid edema
- Conjunctival chemosis
- Proptosis

Management

The Endophthalmitis Vitrectomy Study provides treatment recommendations. This study showed that vitrectomy was unnecessary for eyes with hand motion or better vision. It also showed that intravenous antibiotics were unnecessary.

Initial Decision Making

Check the wound. A dehiscence mandates repair and a tap or biopsy in the operating room. For eyes with hand motion or better vision with an intact surgical wound, the tap or biopsy can be performed in the clinic or operating room. Eyes with vision less than hand motion should have a vitrectomy in the operating room.

Culture Specimens

The following specimens can be cultured on chocolate and Sabourad agar and thioglycolate broth. A Gram stain should also be obtained.

1. Anterior chamber fluid (0.1 ml) with a 27-gauge needle
2. Vitreous specimen (0.1–0.5 ml) obtained with aspiration with a 27- or 25-gauge needle, or with vitreous biopsy with a vitrectomy instrument without an infusion cannula, or at the beginning of a complete pars plana vitrectomy
3. Vitrectomy cassette contents millipore-filtered

Medications

- Intravitreal vancomycin 1.0 mg/0.1 ml
- Intravitreal amikacin 0.4 mg/0.1 ml
- Subconjunctival vancomycin 25.0 mg/0.5 ml
- Subconjunctival ceftazidime 100.0 mg/0.5 ml (amikacin 25.0 mg/0.5 ml if patient is penicillin allergic)
- Subconjunctival dexamethasone 6.00 mg/0.25 ml
- Topical vancomycin 50 mg/ml 1 gtt q8h (q2h if wound abnormality) *alternating with*

- Topical amikacin 20 mg/ml 1 gtt q8h (q2h if wound abnormality)
- Topical 1% atropine or 0.25% scopolamine, 1 gtt q4–12h
- Prednisolone 1% acetate, 1 gtt q1–2h
- Oral prednisone 30 mg PO bid beginning on the first postoperative day

UVEITIS MASQUERADE SYNDROMES

Uveitis masquerade syndrome most commonly refers to a malignancy presenting as uveitis.

Ocular Lymphoma

Large-cell lymphoma in particular is well known to present as "uveitis." The patient is usually older and presents with a painless decrease in vision. The condition is bilateral in 75% of cases. Typically the eye appears quiet with chronic clumps of cells and no flare. There may be multifocal, yellow-white retinal pigment epithelium (RPE) infiltrates or detachments. The patient often has a history of incomplete response to steroids. The long-term prognosis for ocular lymphoma is poor, with a 23% 5-year survival rate.

Workup

- Computed tomography (CT) scan of the central nervous system and whole body
- Lumbar puncture for cytology
- Vitrectomy or vitreous biopsy

Treatment

- Radiation treatment to eye and brain
- Intrathecal methotrexate

Other Masquerade Conditions

- Malignant melanoma
- Retinoblastoma

- Leukemia
- Metastatic carcinoma
- Retinitis pigmentosa
- Retinal detachment
- Retained intraocular foreign body
- Amyloidosis

IRITIS AND IRIDOCYCLITIS

The commonly associated signs and symptoms of acute iridocyclitis (e.g., photophobia, pain, limbal injection, miotic pupil) are well known. It must be stressed, however, that proper diagnosis and management depend on the clinician being able to actually visualize cell or flare, or both.

VISUALIZING CELL AND FLARE

The examiner should position himself or herself behind the slit-lamp using the highest magnification and the brightest light source. The examination room should be darkened and the examiner should allow time to become adapted to the darkness. Using a conical beam or a shortened parallelepiped, the examiner should focus on the cornea and then shift focus slightly forward toward the patient (more posterior). The aqueous can then be viewed using the pupil as a backdrop. Cells appear as individual small, white particles that can be counted. Flare is proteinaceous exudate that appears as a milkiness of the normally optically empty aqueous.

When cells are limited to the anterior chamber, the proper diagnosis is iritis. If cells are also present behind the crystalline lens, iridocyclitis is the correct diagnosis. Cells should be graded using the criteria in Table 6.1.

THERAPY

- Topical steroids are appropriate as initial therapy for most iritis cases.

Table 6.1   Grading and Initial Therapy of Iritis

Grade	Cells/Field[a]	Dosage[b]
Rare	1	qid
Trace	2–5	qid
1+	6–10	q3–4h
2+	11–20	q2–3h
3+	21–50	q1–2h
4+	Too many to count	At least every hour[c]

[a]Field = slit 1 mm wide by 3 mm long.
[b]Dosage refers to 1% prednisolone acetate. A cycloplegic agent such as 5% homatropine 1–3 times a day should also be used in all but the most minor cases of iridocyclitis.
[c]Consideration should be given to an alternate delivery of steroid—e.g., contact lens, periocular injections—for severe cases.

- Cycloplegics (e.g., 5% homatropine or 0.25% scopolamine 1–4 times a day) may be indicated to prevent posterior synechiae and to relieve ciliary spasm.
- Recommendations for initiating therapy are listed in Table 6.1.
- Patients should generally be reevaluated in 3–7 days.
- The dosage may be tapered once there is definite clinical improvement.
- Patients on steroids for more than 1 week should be watched for a secondary rise in intraocular pressure and managed appropriately.
- Patients should also be cautioned not to discontinue their medications abruptly because of a possible recurrence of inflammation.
- Collagen shields soaked in dexamethasone, along with hourly administration of drops, can increase steroid concentration in the anterior chamber without periocular injections.

Stepwise Approach to Medical Therapy

1. Topical steroids
2. Subtenons, transeptal, or retrobulbar steroid injections (e.g., triamcinolone acetate 40 mg)

3. Systemic steroids (e.g., prednisone 80 mg PO qd)
4. Immunosuppressives (mandatory in certain diseases such as Wegener's granulomatosis and Behçet's disease)

Nonsteroidal anti-inflammatory drugs (both oral and topical) are not considered useful as first-line agents but can be beneficial in the treatment of cystoid macular edema. They are also useful for their steroid-sparing effect. For example, oral indomethacin can be used in patients who have frequent relapses of uveitis or who flare up on attempted steroid taper. As always, be cognizant of possible systemic side effects of systemic agents.

Special Considerations

Many patients with chronic iritis show few symptoms. There may be no redness or pain. The grading system is especially useful in managing these cases.

It is important to perform a careful dilated fundus examination in patients with anterior uveitis, because a certain number of these patients will also present with a posterior uveitis.

Key Points

- A myriad of systemic disorders can be associated with iritis.
- Infrequently, medications can be the cause of iritis.
- Laboratory studies are not indicated unless the uveitis has unusual features, is unresponsive to standard therapy or is recurrent, or when symptoms or signs of an associated condition are present.
- Some thought as to the most likely diagnoses must be given before ancillary studies are ordered to minimize unnecessary testing. Only after considering demographic factors, asking about specific symptoms, and completing the ocular examination can these studies be ordered with a sense of purpose.
- Table 6.2 is intended as a useful guide when ancillary studies are contemplated.

Table 6.2 Common Uveitic Syndromes

Type/Location	Notes	Special Tests
Idiopathic, A, P	Most common cause of anterior uveitis	None
Ankylosing spondylitis, A	More common in males; may give history of lower back pain	Spine and pelvic x-rays, HLA-B27, ESR, rheumatology consultation
Inflammatory bowel, A	May also find uveitis with enteritis, Crohn's, or Whipple's disease	Medical consultation, gastrointestinal x-rays, intestinal biopsy, HLA-B27
Juvenile rheumatoid arthritis, A	Most often found in young females; pauciarticular arthritis	Antinuclear antibody, ESR, HLA-B8, rheumatology consultation
Reiter's syndrome, A	Most often found in men with history of venereal disease. Often show triad of conjunctivitis, urethritis, arthritis. Also seen with gram-negative dysentery.	HLA-B27, ESR, sacroiliac x-ray, DFA or culture for chlamydia
Heterochromatic cyclitis, A	Involved iris is usually lighter with stromal atrophy; iris neovascularization is a potential complication; treat iritis only when severe	None
Phakoanaphylaxis, A	Uveitis secondary to lens protein; seen after cataract surgery or trauma; surgical removal of lens material often necessary.	None

Table 6.2 (continued)

Type/Location	Notes	Special Tests
Herpes simplex, A, rarely P	Most often seen along with herpes stromal keratitis; antiviral agents with steroids may be required	Usually none required; can do DFA or CF if questionable
Herpes zoster, A	Seen in association with "shingles"; may also see corneal involvement, trabeculitis, glaucoma, ocular motor palsies, and, rarely, optic neuritis	None
Pars planitis, A, P	Cells in anterior vitreous; "snow banking" of peripheral retina or over pars plana; often bilateral	Consider MRI; rule out MS; consider Lyme titers
Sarcoid, A, P	Most often seen in blacks; may see "candle wax drippings" with posterior segments	Chest x-ray, conjunctival biopsy, ACE, gallium scan, internal medicine consultation
Tuberculosis, A, P	Should be suspected in any granulomatous uveitis of anterior or posterior segments	PPD (skin test), chest x-ray, medical consultation
Syphilis, A, P	Acquired syphilis may show iritis, vitritis, choroiditis, or optic neuritis	FTA-ABS, VDRL, lumbar puncture, HIV serology, medical consultation
Toxoplasmosis, A, P	May see retinitis; vitritis often with reactivation from old chorioretinal scar	ELISA for toxoplasmosis

Toxocariasis, A, P	Active lesions most often seen in young children as large retinal granuloma with vitreal strands	ELISA titer if diagnosis in doubt
Vogt-Koyanagi-Harada syndrome, A, P	Seen most often in Asians and Native Americans; alopecia, vitiligo, poliosis, hearing problems, granulomatous panuveitis	Audiometry, lumbar puncture, MRI
Behçet's syndrome, A, P	Usually Asian or Mediterranean men 20–40 years old; uveitis often with hypopyon; aphthous mouth lesions and genital ulcers	HLA-B5, medical consult
Sympathetic ophthalmia, A, P	Bilateral panuveitis seen after trauma to *one* eye	None
Cytomegalovirus, P	Extensive hemorrhage; necrotic retinitis seen in immunocompromised	Diagnosis is clinical. Can get urine and sputum culture, serology
"Birdshot" chorioretinopathy, P	Bilateral low-grade vasculitis often becoming severe	HLA-A29*
Histoplasmosis, P	Small punched-out chorioretinal scars; peripapillary atrophy; choroidal neovascular membranes. Most common in Midwest	None usually; histoplasmin skin test may reactivate; chest x-ray rarely needed.

Table 6.2   (continued)

Type/Location	Notes	Special Tests
AMPPPE, P, occasionally A	Cream-colored placoid lesions of pigment epithelium; usually aged 15–40 yrs; resolves without treatment.	None
Multifocal choroiditis, P	Pseudohistoplasmosis picture; more common in females; usually bilateral retinochoroiditis and vitritis associated with elevated Epstein-Barr virus serology	Epstein-Barr virus serology
Geographic (serpiginous) choroiditis, P	Cream-colored helicoid choroiditis usually radiating from optic disc	None
Cytomegalic inclusion, P	Retinitis or retinochoroiditis can be seen in AIDS	Virus studies of urine, serum, CF test
Acute retinal necrosis and PORN, P	Etiology is herpes simplex zoster virus. Treatment may include acyclovir and aspirin	Consider polymerase chain reaction study for herpes zoster virus and herpes simplex virus

A = anterior uveitis; P = posterior uveitis; HLA = human leukocyte antigen; ESR = erythrocyte sedimentation rate; DFA = direct fluorescent antibody; CF = complement fixation; MRI = magnetic resonance imaging; MS = multiple sclerosis; ACE = angiotensin-converting enzyme; PPD = purified protein derivative; FTA-ABS = fluorescent treponemal antibody absorption; VDRL = Venereal Disease Research Laboratory; HIV = human immunodeficiency virus; ELISA = enzyme-linked immunosorbent assay; CMV = cytomegalovirus; AMPPPE = acute multifocal posterior placoid pigment epitheliopathy.
*These are generally not "first-line" tests.

7

Episcleritis and Scleritis

EPISCLERITIS

Episcleritis is characterized by diffuse or segmental inflammation of the episclera. Symptoms are generally minimal. Usually there is no discharge and patients complain of only mild photophobia, burning, or lacrimation. When the inflammation is localized and of sufficient intensity, nodular episcleritis may result. The disease is characterized by multiple recurrences.

Diagnosis

Episcleritis is distinguished from conjunctivitis by the depth of vascular engorgement. Episcleral vessels will not move when the conjunctiva is mechanically moved by applying pressure with a finger through the lid. The application of topical phenylephrine is another method to distinguish conjunctivitis from episcleritis. Phenylephrine will blanch conjunctival vessels but will have little effect on the deeper episcleral vessels.

Management

Episcleritis is a benign disorder that usually resolves without treatment in 10–21 days. Symptomatic relief and faster resolution can be obtained through the use of topical steroids. The recurrent nature of the disease should be kept in mind, however. Patients can become heavily dependent on steroids and thus become unnecessarily exposed to the harmful side effects.

For mild attacks, supportive measures such as cold compresses and the use of topical vasoconstrictors may be the best approach. Prednisolone acetate 1% or fluorometholone 0.1% applied 4–6 times a day and gradually tapered over 1–2 weeks may be justified in more severe cases.

Unless the patient has specific systemic symptoms or an unusually severe or recalcitrant episode, a search for the underlying associated medical disorders is not indicated. About 15% of cases are associated with collagen vascular disease, prior herpes zoster ophthalmicus, or gout.

SCLERITIS

In contrast to episcleritis, scleritis can result in permanent vision-threatening sequelae. A deep boring pain is often associated with this condition, and the engorged vessels may take on a bluish or violet hue, unlike the bright red pattern of injection seen in episcleritis. The most common types of scleritis are diffuse anterior and nodular anterior scleritis. Posterior scleritis may be associated with reduced visual acuity, proptosis, lid retraction, and choroidal or exudative retinal detachment. The most severe form of scleritis is necrotizing scleritis, which is characterized by focal areas of avascular scleral dropout and transparency. Eventually the underlying uvea can become exposed and result in perforation of the globe. The majority of patients with necrotizing scleritis have an underlying collagen vascular or vasculitic disease. Topical drugs are insufficient for treatment of scleritis. *Subconjunctival steroid injections are contraindicated because of the potential risk of scleral perforation.*

Associated Conditions

- Rheumatoid arthritis
- Wegener's granulomatosis
- Relapsing polychondritis
- Systemic lupus erythematosus
- Inflammatory bowel disease
- Reiter's syndrome

Management of Diffuse and Nodular Scleritis

1. First-line treatment:
   - Sustained-release indomethacin 75 mg PO bid, *or*
   - Diflunisal 500 mg PO bid
2. For therapeutic failures, try different nonsteroidal anti-inflammatory drugs (NSAIDs) in succession. For example:
   - Naproxen 500 mg bid, *or*
   - Ibuprofen 400–600 mg bid, *or*
   - Sulindac 200 mg bid
3. If NSAID therapy fails, add:
   - Prednisone 60–120 mg/day for 1 week with rapid tapering to 20 mg/day for 2–3 weeks
   - Maintain remission with NSAIDs
4. Immunosuppressive drugs for recalcitrant cases (the last three can be used alone or in combination):
   - Methotrexate 7.5–15.0 mg PO or 15 mg IM once a week
   - Cyclophosphamide 1–2 mg/kg per day PO, *or*
   - Azathioprine 1–2 mg/kg per day PO, *or*
   - Cyclosporine 3–5 mg/kg per day PO

Management of Necrotizing Scleritis

First-line agents are immunosuppressants.

- Cyclophosphamide 1–2 mg/kg per day PO
- Other choices can be found under diffuse and nodular scleritis (above).

NOTES

8

Vision Loss

UNEXPLAINED VISION LOSS

The investigation of unexplained visual acuity loss begins with a careful history and review of medications and health status. If the physician is unable to uncover the cause of the visual acuity loss in a standard examination (e.g., refraction, keratometry, slit-lamp, ophthalmoscopy), he or she should try to determine the characteristics of the loss (e.g., central scotoma, caecocentral scotoma) with visual field testing, Amsler grid testing, and color-vision testing before resorting to more invasive or elaborate testing such as fluorescein angiography and radiologic tests.

In unilateral cases of visual acuity loss, careful attention should be paid to the fellow eye when testing the visual fields. A temporal field defect in the asymptomatic eye may direct the clinician to consider a chiasmal lesion, for example.

Testing with the red Amsler grid can be especially helpful in picking up subtle central field defects in early optic nerve disease such as nutritional amblyopia.

Color-vision testing is less reliable in differentiating between macular and optic nerve disease than the photostress test. In general, optic nerve disease results in red-green defects and macular disease results in blue-yellow defects, but exceptions to this rule are not too uncommon. In addition, it should be kept in mind that even mild unilateral or asymmetric optic nerve disease generally results in a Marcus Gunn pupil, whereas only substantial retinal disease will result in an afferent pupillary defect (see the section on Marcus Gunn sign in Chapter 10). Consideration should always be given to the possibility of functional vision loss.

Photostress Test

Measure the amount of time needed for a patient to read the line on the visual acuity chart above the lowest line read after shining a light source (ophthalmoscope) into the eye for 10 seconds. For example, if a patient's best corrected acuity is 20/40, how long does it take the patient to recover from the ophthalmoscope light to read the 20/50 line? Compare this to the fellow eye. The recovery time is generally greatly prolonged in macular disease.

Often-Missed Causes of Visual Acuity Loss

- Milky-white nuclear sclerotic cataract
- Keratoconus
- Nutritional (tobacco-alcohol) amblyopia
- Toxic amblyopia
- Preexisting amblyopia
- Leber's optic neuropathy (optic nerve changes may be quite subtle—hyperemia, telangiectasia)
- Stargardt's disease (visual acuity loss may precede obvious fundus changes)
- Retrobulbar optic neuritis (patient should have Marcus Gunn pupil)
- Retrobulbar or subtle anterior ischemic optic neuropathy
- Macular cyst
- Macular edema (as in diabetic retinopathy, cystoid edema in aphakia, or pars planitis)
- Central serous maculopathy
- Retrobulbar or intracranial mass
- Hysteria
- Malingering

MALINGERING AND HYSTERICAL AMBLYOPIA

Malingering and hysterical amblyopia are both nonorganic or functional causes of apparent visual acuity loss. The difference is that the malingerer makes an effort to feign visual loss, usually for some personal gain. The hysterical amblyope, on the other hand, has a subconscious origin for his or her visual loss. The patient is unaware that his or her vision problem is psychogenic.

Proving that both of these groups of patients are capable of good visual function can be challenging, to say the least, and a certain amount of suspicion is important in coming up with the correct diagnosis. Malingerers may be somewhat easier to identify in that they often exaggerate their visual dysfunction and may be less cooperative during testing. Hysterical amblyopes, on the other hand, tend to be cooperative and function at a much better level than would be expected from visual acuity measurements. Other tip-offs that should alert the physician to the possibility of functional vision loss include:

- Unequal distance and near visual acuities
- Ability to subjectively differentiate between small changes in lens power/axis during refraction
- Disproportionately large increases in visual acuity from small lens changes during refraction

Once the clinician thinks he or she is dealing with a functional disorder, the examination should be geared toward proving this by demonstrating good acuity. This is also important to protect both the doctor and the patient from possible mislabeling of an organic problem. The following tests may be useful in this regard:

1. Visual fields: The individual with functional vision loss may show peripheral contracture of the visual fields. The visual field may be tubular—i.e., the visual field will have the same width when plotted on a tangent screen at both 1 and 2 meters. Other possibilities are spiraling inward of the field on repeated testing or very irregular isopters.
2. Optokinetic nystagmus: Involuntary optokinetic nystagmus movements to a drum or flag indicate at least some gross visual function.
3. Menace or blink reflex: Indicates at least gross visual function
4. Three-card test: Show patient two cards with nondescript words

(e.g., dog, cat) using the eye in question. The third card contains a vulgarity. After showing this card, the patient is observed for an appropriate response.

The following tests are useful for monocular decreased acuity only:

5. Four base-out test: A four-diopter base-out prism placed in front of an eye with poor vision will yield no movement of the fellow eye because of a lack of fusion. If fusion is present, the fellow eye will show an adducting movement.
6. Unequal binocular plus: Behind the phoropter and with neither eye occluded, the doctor slips a +3.00 lens in front of the fellow eye. Ability to obtain good visual acuity is proof that the eye in question is capable of good visual function.
7. AO vectographic slides: With both eyes open and the patient wearing analyzers, the patient is asked to read the vectographic slide chart. This can also be accomplished with the patient wearing red/green lenses and viewing the projector chart with the red/green filter used for binocular balance.

NOTES

9

Pediatric Ophthalmology

AMBLYOPIA

Amblyopia is usually a term used to describe a developmental cause of vision deficiency not adequately explained by an organic lesion. If vision does not develop properly during the crucial first few years of life and if treatment or correction is not offered, this may lead to a permanent visual disability.

Etiologies

- Anisometropia
- Astigmatism
- Strabismus
- Media opacity and occlusion (e.g., congenital cataract, ptosis)

Treatment

- Correct the cause of occlusion if known (e.g., cataract surgery).
- Correct refractive error with spectacles.
- Occlude the preferred eye (one with better visual acuity) with an adhesive patch. Schedule of patching may be based on the patient's age. Examples:
  1. Alternate patching in 3:1 ratio during first year of life (occlude the sound eye for 3 days followed by occlusion of the amblyopic eye)
  2. The ratio may be 4:1 or 5:1 for 2- to 4-year-old children.
  3. Full-time occlusion without alternation in children 5–11 years of age

4. There is usually little benefit in patching children older than 12 years of age.
- Follow up at monthly intervals. Discontinue patching once visual acuity stabilizes on three successive visits or until acuity of the amblyopic eye is equal to the fellow eye.

ESOTROPIA IN CHILDREN

Etiologies

1. Nonconcomitant deviations
   - Sixth nerve palsy—the angle of deviation changes with the position of gaze. (See the following section on diplopia and cranial nerve palsies.)
2. Concomitant deviations
   - Congenital esotropia (present by 6 months of age)
   - Accommodative esotropia (due to hyperopia and convergence that results from accommodating)
   - Sensory deprivation (seen with organic cause of reduced vision)
   - Divergence insufficiency

Management of Concomitant Esotropias

- Differentiate concomitant esotropias from pseudoesotropia (due to wide bridge, epicanthal folds, etc.). Pseudoesotropias will show no tropia on cover test.
- Perform cycloplegic refraction.
- Prescription is indicated for significant hyperopia (>2.00 D). Consider executive bifocals fit to the bottom edge of the pupils if esotropia is greater at near vision.
- Occlusion therapy is indicated for suspected amblyopia (see preceding section on amblyopia).
- Consider orthoptics/vision therapy for low-angle esotropia that may remain.
- Muscle surgery may be indicated for significant esotropia not corrected by spectacles and too great for vision therapy after therapy

for amblyopia. There is still some disagreement about optimal age; usually it is between 6 months and 2 years of age.

VERTICAL DEVIATIONS

Dissociated Vertical Deviation

- Characterized by the upward drifting of an occluded or nonfixating eye during periods of visual inattention
- Differs from a hypertropia or hyperphoria in that when the upward deviated eye returns to a horizontal position, there is no corrective downward movement in the fellow eye
- Seen commonly in congenital esotropia
- Treatment indicated only if it occurs frequently and is cosmetically significant

Double Elevator Palsy

- Characterized by hypotropia of the involved eye that increases in upward gaze
- Limited elevation of the involved eye on versions and ductions both in abduction and adduction
- May be associated with inferior rectus muscle restriction
- Ptosis or pseudoptosis is often present.
- Patients may present in a chin-up position.
- Patients may present with a deep extra lower-lid fold.
- Patients often present with a poor Bell's phenomenon on the involved side.

Management

- For restricted inferior rectus: recession of the inferior rectus
- If there is no restriction, a Knapp procedure may be performed (transposition of the medial and lateral recti toward the superior rectus).

Brown's Syndrome (Superior Oblique Tendon Sheath Syndrome)

- Characterized by limited elevation of the involved eye only in adduction
- There may be depression of the involved eye in adduction.
- Forced duction testing is positive.
- There is an exotropia on upgaze.

Management

- Avoid surgery if possible. Surgery is reserved for significant cosmetic disfigurement from head tilts or large hypodeviations.

RETINOPATHY OF PREMATURITY

Retinopathy of prematurity (ROP) is a vasoproliferative retinal disorder occurring in premature and low-birth-weight infants often associated with supplemental oxygen administration. It may progress and lead to total retinal detachment and blindness. It is important to detect and treat ROP in a timely manner.

Infants at Risk

- Birth weight less than 1,500 g
- Gestational age less than 28 weeks
- The necessity for supplemental oxygen further increases the risk.

Grading

The grading of retinopathy involves staging the severity as well as describing the location of these changes.

Staging

Stage 1: A demarcation line
Stage 2: A ridge
Stage 3: A ridge with extraretinal fibrovascular proliferation
Stage 4: Subtotal retinal detachment
Stage 4A: Extrafoveal retinal detachment

Stage 4B: Retinal detachment involving the fovea
Stage 5: Total retinal detachment
Plus disease: Severe vascular shunting with enlarged veins and tortuous arterioles in the posterior pole

Location

Zone I: A circle of 30-degree radius (twice the disc to macula distance) centered at the optic disc
Zone II: From the edge of zone I to the nasal ora serrata and around to an area near the temporal equator
Zone III: The residual temporal crescent anterior to zone II (Fig. 9.1)

Management

The first retinal examination is generally performed 4–6 weeks after birth. Subsequent exams are performed at intervals dictated by the degree of retinopathy (Fig. 9.2).

- The recommended solution for pupil dilation and cycloplegia is Cyclomydril (cyclopentolate 0.2% and phenylephrine 1%).
- Laser photocoagulation is offered if retinopathy reaches threshold (see the section on threshold disease below).
- Scleral buckling and vitrectomy may be used to treat stage 5 disease.
- Screening fundus examinations can be discontinued once the retina is fully vascularized (vessels 1 disc diameter from the nasal ora).

Threshold Disease

Threshold disease is characterized by stage 3+ disease in zone I or II involving (1) at least five contiguous clock-hour sectors or (2) at least eight interrupted clock-hour sectors.

ANIRIDIA

Aniridia is a bilateral disorder that may be a familial form (in which case it is inherited in an autosomal dominant fashion) or may be a sporadic form that can be associated with Wilms' tumor or the ARG

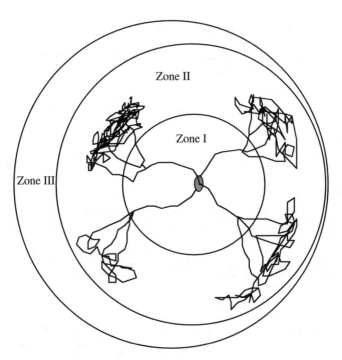

Fig. 9.1   The grading of retinopathy depends on an assessment of the stage and location of retinal abnormalities.

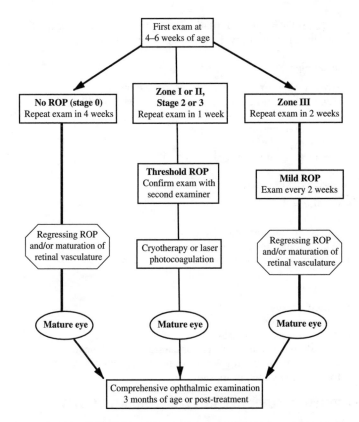

Fig. 9.2 Flow diagram for following retinopathy of prematurity (ROP) based on American Academy of Ophthalmology. Basic and Clinical Science Course. Section 6, 1996–1997. San Francisco: American Academy of Ophthalmology, 1997.

triad (aniridia, mental retardation, and genitourinary abnormalities). Clinically, a rudimentary iris can usually be found.

Clinical Signs

- Absent irides or very large, unresponsive pupils
- Edge of lens and ciliary processes visible without dilation
- Photophobia
- Congenital sensory nystagmus
- Foveal hypoplasia
- Subnormal vision (20/100 or worse)

Associated Abnormalities

- Cataracts
- Glaucoma
- Persistent pupillary membranes
- Wilms' tumor in sporadic form
- ARG triad (see above) in sporadic form

Management

- Tinted glasses
- Low vision aids
- Prosthetic contact lenses
- Periodic eye exams to check for cataracts and glaucoma
- Periodic evaluation for Wilms' tumor (ultrasound or computed tomography scans) in sporadic cases

UVEITIS IN JUVENILE RHEUMATOID ARTHRITIS

Juvenile rheumatoid arthritis (JRA) is associated with a severe and insidious vision loss from anterior uveitis. It is painless and appears in a white eye that, on external exam, appears uninflamed.

The forms of JRA most commonly associated with iridocyclitis are the following:

1. The pauciarticular early-onset form seen most commonly in young girls. Sixty percent have antinuclear antibodies (ANAs), and the rheumatoid factor (RF) tends to be negative.
2. The pauciarticular form seen more commonly in somewhat older males (onset after 8 years of age). These patients tend to be both RF negative and ANA negative. The majority are HLA-B27 negative. These patients may have a tendency to develop ankylosing spondylitis, Reiter's syndrome, or inflammatory bowel disease.

Management

- Frequent ophthalmic examinations (see examination schedule)
- Aspirin, 100 mg/kg/day
- Topical steroids and cycloplegic agents during active uveitis
- Systemic steroids (2 mg/kg/day of prednisone) during severe exacerbations
- Monitor for evidence of glaucoma, cataracts, and band keratopathy.

CONGENITAL CATARACTS

Routine pediatric care is indicated in healthy children with unilateral cataracts, but if the cataract is bilateral, a medical workup to determine its cause may be indicated (Table 9.1).

Treatment

- Evaluate pupil, optic nerve, retina, and so forth for visual potential.
- Some less significant opacities may be treated with pupil dilation and occlusion therapy as needed.
- Cataract surgery should be performed during the first 6–8 weeks of life for visually significant opacities. A posterior capsulotomy and anterior vitrectomy should be performed at the time of surgery
- Contact lens correction and aggressive amblyopia therapy are indicated in most cases of congenital cataract.

Table 9.1   Routine Screening in Children with Bilateral Cataracts

Test	Disorder
Chromosome analysis	Down syndrome and other disorders
Examination of parents, siblings	Hereditary cataracts
Serum calcium	Hypoparathyroidism
TORCH titers	Toxoplasmosis, rubella, cyto-megalovirus, herpes
Urine amino acids	Lowe syndrome
Urine-reducing substances	Galactosemia

SHAKEN BABY SYNDROME

The term shaken baby syndrome refers to the constellation of clini-cal findings that may occur when an abused infant is violently shaken. Often there is no bruising or other outward signs of trauma. A dilated fundus examination in an infant with unexplained neuro-logic injury or abnormalities can confirm the diagnosis.

Signs and Symptoms

- Child under 2 years of age
- Seizure, lethargy, loss of consciousness, respiratory arrest, vomiting
- Subdural or other intracranial injury on neuroimaging
- Retinal hemorrhages, vitreous hemorrhage, and cotton-wool spots (retinal hemorrhages that result from the birthing process resolve by 4 weeks of age)
- Retinal detachment and retinoschisis
- Papilledema

Management

The physician does not need to determine who is responsible for the injury, but the reporting of suspected cases of child abuse is man-dated by all 50 states. The hospital social worker should be involved early in the case. Treatment may include retinal reattachment surgery or vitrectomy for nonclearing vitreous hemorrhage.

CONGENITAL GLAUCOMA

Signs and Symptoms

- Corneal edema often is the presenting sign in infants. Corneal edema may be microcystic or stromal. Breaks in Descemet's membrane (Haab's striae) may develop, leading to high degrees of astigmatism.
- Corneal enlargement. The average horizontal corneal diameter in newborns is 9.5 mm. At 2 years of age, the average horizontal corneal diameter is 11.5 mm.
- Tearing and photophobia
- Myopia, which is a result of enlargement of the eye from high pressure
- Enlarged cup-to-disc ratio. Enlargement of the cup may be reversed with normalization of intraocular pressure.
- Increased intraocular pressure (IOP). Measurement of IOP can sometimes be accomplished in the office with a hand-held tonometer while the infant is sleeping or feeding from a bottle. It should be kept in mind that most anesthetics (with the exception of ketamine) lower IOP.

Management

Immediate surgery is the appropriate therapy, most commonly with goniotomy or trabeculotomy. Trabeculectomy, often with mitomycin, may be necessary if goniotomy or trabeculotomy cannot be accomplished. Surgical implants or ciliary body ablation procedures may be necessary when more conservative surgical procedures fail.

Medical therapy may be used briefly until surgery can be arranged and on occasion adjunctively if target IOPs are not met after surgery. Carbonic anhydrase inhibitors, beta blockers, miotics, and prostaglandins have all been used.

Amblyopia may be the biggest threat to vision. Aggressive therapy is often necessary.

RETINOBLASTOMA

Retinoblastoma is the most common intraocular tumor of childhood. Approximately 5–10% of patients have a family history of retinoblastoma. In approximately two-thirds of patients, the tumor is monocular. In about one-third of patients, the tumor results from a germinal mutation, and multiple bilateral tumors may result. Retinoblastoma is typically diagnosed during the first year of life in familial and bilateral cases. Most unilateral, sporadic cases are diagnosed between 1 and 3 years of age.

Signs and Symptoms

- Leukocoria (white pupil)
- Strabismus
- White or cream-colored calcified mass with or without tortuous large-caliber vessels
- Vitreous hemorrhage and hyphema are less common presenting signs.
- Vitreous seeding can result in a clinical picture that resembles endophthalmitis.
- In advanced cases, retinoblastoma can have an orbital presentation with progressive proptosis, lid swelling, and ecchymoses.

Management

Intraocular retinoblastoma can be treated successfully with a 90% 5-year survival rate. The prognosis for patients with orbital extension, however, remains grim, and 90% succumb to their disease.

- Enucleation is the mainstay of therapy in most instances.
- External beam irradiation, brachytherapy, cryotherapy, or photocoagulation can be used in an effort to salvage one globe in bilateral cases or in unilateral cases with an early diagnosis.

- Chemotherapy is playing a role in the management at some treatment centers.
- A metastatic workup, including cerebrospinal fluid examination, bone marrow examination, bone scan, and chest x-ray if there is evidence of extraocular disease or significant optic nerve or choroidal invasion, should be performed.
- A genetic workup including evaluation of other family members should be performed.
- Retinoblastoma patients with the germinal mutation should be carefully monitored for the development of intracranial tumors (especially pineal gland), osteosarcomas, and soft-tissue sarcomas.

NOTES

10

Pupil and Acquired Oculomotor Abnormalities

EPISODIC ANISOCORIA

Anisocoria is not commonly found to be intermittent in nature and thus is often more of a challenge for the clinician.

Intermittent Dilation

Parasympathetic Paresis

- Uncal herniation (other signs present)
- Seizure disorders
- Migraine

Sympathetic Hyperactivity

- Claude Bernard syndrome, which is secondary to neck trauma. Patients also have headaches, lid retraction, and hyperhidrosis.

Benign Pupillary Dilation

- Patients may have associated headache but no other neurologic signs. Pupils react briskly during periods of dilation.

Note: The possibility of aneurysm should be considered in all cases of pupillary dilation. Patients with isolated, intermittent pupil dilation should be monitored regularly.

Intermittent Constriction

Parasympathetic Hyperactivity

• Parasympathetic spasm; only one case has been reported.

Sympathetic Paresis

• Horner's syndrome from cluster headache

CONSTANT ANISOCORIA

The following pages can be used in the evaluation of a patient with anisocoria. Alternatively, the flow charts in Figs. 10.1 and 10.2 can be used in arriving at a correct diagnosis.

The pupil sizes should be checked in both dim and bright illumination. The briskness of the pupil's response to light should be assessed using a cool, bright light source while the patient is fixating on a distant object. If the response is slow or absent, refer to the section on abnormal light reaction below.

Normal Light Reaction

Compare the difference in pupil size at 5 and 10 seconds under dim illumination after shining a bright light into the eyes for a few seconds.

• Physiologic anisocoria: Anisocoria is equal under dim and bright illumination, and there is no difference in anisocoria at 5 or 10 seconds.
• Horner's syndrome: Anisocoria is greater at 5 than at 10 seconds. Also, it is more pronounced under dim illumination. Do a cocaine test if in doubt. (See the section on Horner's syndrome below.)

Sluggish or No Light Reaction

Once it has been determined that the pupil response to light is abnormal, the response to near vision should be checked by having the patient fixate on his or her finger or other near object for several seconds. The patient should then fixate on a distant object, and the physician should watch for dilation.

Anisocoria greatest in dim light

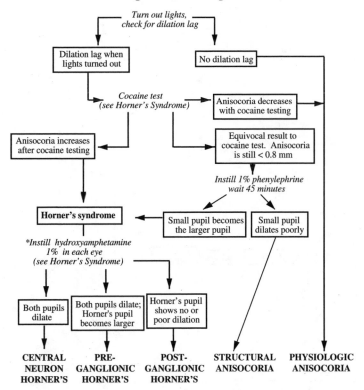

Fig. 10.1 The identification of Horner's syndrome is the key in evaluating patients with anisocoria that increases in dim illumination. Note: An "old" Adie's pupil may be smaller than the normal pupil and dilate poorly, thus presenting with greater inequality in the dark.

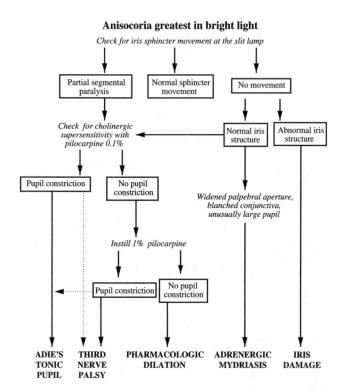

Fig. 10.2   Identification of cholinergic sensitivity or resistance to miotic agents is the key to sorting out an anisocoria that increases in bright light. Note: Cholinergic sensitivity takes a few days to develop in Adie's pupil. A third nerve palsy may demonstrate some cholinergic sensitivity. A third nerve palsy should demonstrate other signs (ptosis, motility disturbance). (Adapted from HS Thompson, SFJ Pilley. Unequal pupils. A flow chart for sorting out the anibocorias. Surv Ophthalmol 1976;21(1):45–48.)

Normal Near Response

Pupils that show a greater response to accommodation than to light are said to show light-near dissociation. The causes are listed below:

- Midbrain lesion. Usually the pupils are dilated bilaterally. The lesion may be associated with superior gaze palsy. Magnetic resonance imaging (MRI) may be indicated.
- Syphilis (usually small pupils)
- Advanced juvenile diabetes
- Chronic alcoholism
- Aberrant regeneration of third nerve
- Adie's tonic pupil (usually sluggish to near)

Sluggish or No Near Response

- Trauma, synechiae, or high intraocular pressure
- Adie's tonic pupil (benign); larger pupil often in women ages 20–40. Iris streaming may be noted under slit lamp. Reacts to ⅛% pilocarpine.
- Pharmacologic (as from dilating drops, etc.). Pupil shows no response to 1% pilocarpine.
- Third-nerve lesion. Pupil will react to 1% pilocarpine, but this test is rarely necessary. Usually the lesion is associated with ptosis and oculomotor palsy.

HORNER'S SYNDROME

Horner's syndrome is due to a lesion of the sympathetic innervation to the eye. It is characterized clinically by relative miosis and lid ptosis on the involved side, both of which may be very subtle and easily missed during a cursory examination. It is important to follow through in making the diagnosis and localizing the lesion once the disorder is suspected because it may have life-threatening implications. The exception, of course, is congenital Horner's syndrome as a result of birth trauma. Many of these cases will show heterochromia iridis (lighter iris in the involved eye) or can easily be confirmed by viewing old photographs.

Diagnosis

- Dilation lag: Because of relative weakness of the dilator, after a bright light or flash is presented to the eyes, the anisocoria of Horner's syndrome is greater 5 seconds after presentation than at 10 seconds. This test should be performed in dim light with the patient fixating on a distant target.
- Cocaine test should be performed if dilation lag is equivocal. Instill 1 drop of 10% cocaine in each eye. The test must be done before any procedure that might disrupt the corneal epithelium. The fellow pupil is observed as the control. A normal pupil will dilate from cocaine; the Horner's eye will not. If after 40 minutes neither pupil dilates, instill another drop and wait. A positive test (no or very little dilation of the pupil in question) should cause the clinician to determine whether the location of the lesion is pre- or postganglionic (see below).

Pre- vs. Postganglionic Horner's Syndrome

Children with Horner's syndrome require further investigation, including radiologic studies to rule out malignancy. The exception, again, are those cases that resulted from birth trauma.

Adults with a new case of Horner's syndrome are much more likely to harbor a malignancy if the lesion is preganglionic (first or second neuron). Isolated postganglionic Horner's syndrome is generally benign.

The workup of a Horner's pupil may include a thorough physical examination, a complete blood cell count with differential, cervical x-rays and chest x-rays (for Pancoast's tumor of lungs), and computed tomography or MRI of the brain, depending on the suspected location of the lesion. The tests ordered depend on whether the syndrome is pre- or postganglionic.

Determine pre- versus postganglionic lesions by instilling one drop of 1% hydroxyamphetamine in each eye. The normal fellow pupil should dilate. After 45 minutes the Horner's pupil should show:

- No dilation, meaning it is a postganglionic lesion, *or*
- Dilation, meaning it is a preganglionic lesion (consider lung cancer, brain tumor, stroke, etc.)

MARCUS GUNN SIGN

The swinging flashlight test is extremely useful in differentiating optic nerve from retinal causes of vision loss, because minor optic nerve defects typically produce an afferent pupillary defect (Marcus Gunn sign), whereas only extensive retinal disease is likely to produce the Marcus Gunn sign (Figs. 10.3 and 10.4).

The detection of subtle afferent pupillary defects can be facilitated by the use of neutral density filters alternately placed in front of each eye while performing the swinging flashlight test. For instance, a 0.3 log unit filter placed in front of an eye with minimal optic nerve damage might produce a marked Marcus Gunn sign. The same filter, when placed in front of the fellow "good" eye, may produce no clinically recognizable pupillary defect.

ACUTE-ONSET DIPLOPIA

Patients who describe the sudden onset of double vision require careful investigation, because the source of diplopia may be a life-threatening disorder. After a careful history detailing known health problems, current medications, prior trauma, and other neurologic symptoms, the clinician should gear his or her examination toward determining the etiology of the patient's complaints.

Monocular Diplopia/Polyopia

Patients whose complaints of multiple images are not relieved by occlusion of the fellow eye most often have a refractive or ocular media (e.g., cataract) abnormality. Causes of monocular polyopia include:

- Lens abnormality (e.g., vacuole)
- Irregular astigmatism
- Incorrect correction of refractive error

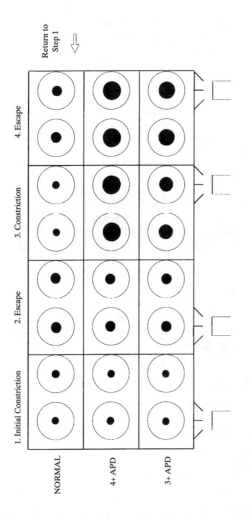

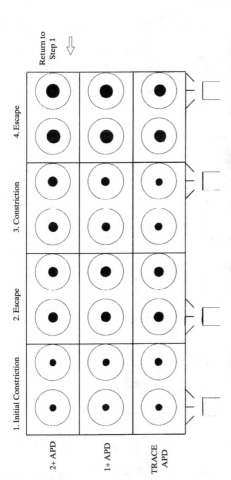

Fig. 10.3   Testing for an afferent pupillary defect (APD). The normal reaction is shown in the *top row*. An afferent defect is found by comparing the pupil's reaction to the fellow eye. Here the left pupil (as seen by the examiner) demonstrates different degrees of defect.

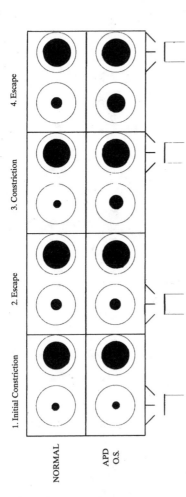

Fig. 10.4 The inverse Marcus Gunn Sign. The right pupil must be observed throughout testing because the left pupil is fixed. In the second row, an afferent defect manifests as less constriction when the light is switched from the right to the left eye. Swinging the flashlight back to the right eye (step 4, then back to step 1) results in a telltale brisk constriction of the right eye.

- Subluxed lens
- Viewing through edge of bifocal or lens
- Peripheral iridectomy/double pupil
- Partial closure of lids (impinging on cornea)
- Looking through edge of intraocular lens
- Vitreal/aqueous abnormalities/opacities
- Retinal detachment
- Macular edema
- Malingering or hysteria
- Systemic or neurologic causes (rare)

Binocular Diplopia

Once the diplopia is confirmed as binocular, it should then be established whether the double vision is horizontal or vertical. It is useful to determine in which position of gaze the angle of deviation is maximal. This is determined by performing cover testing in various positions of gaze. An alternative method is to have the patient view a pen light in different positions of gaze while holding a red lens over the right eye. The patient is then asked to describe the separation of the two images. When a single muscle is involved, the separation of the images is maximal when the light source is moved into the field of the paretic muscle. The involved eye is determined by asking the patient, "Which light is farther away, the red or the white?"

Park's three-step test is useful in isolating vertical muscle paresis. The test can be performed by neutralizing the angle with a prism test while having the patient view a distant target and performing a cover test (Table 10.1).

Etiology of Binocular Diplopia

Most often the etiology of sudden binocular diplopia is a cranial nerve palsy. Obviously one should try to verify that one is indeed dealing with a new palsy. Occasionally a patient is able to compensate for a congenital palsy through head turning or tilting. Old pho-

Table 10.1   Park's Three-Step Technique for Isolating a Paretic Extraocular Muscle

Step 1: Is the patient a right (R) or left (L) hypertrope?
Step 2: Does the deviation increase in gaze right or left?
Step 3: Does the deviation increase with head tilt right or left?

Step 1	Step 2	Step 3	Paretic muscle
R	R	R	LIO
R	R	L	RIR
R	L	R	RSO
R	L	L	LSR
L	R	R	RSR
L	R	L	LSO
L	L	R	LIR
L	L	L	RIO

Example: Right hypertropia, which increases in gaze left and head tilt right = right superior oblique.
LIO = left inferior oblique; RIR = right inferior rectus; RSO = right superior oblique; LSR = left superior rectus; RSR = right superior rectus; LSO = left superior oblique; LIR = left inferior rectus; RIO = right inferior oblique.

tographs are helpful in uncovering this. Other common causes of binocular diplopia and differential features are listed below:

- Decompensated phoria. Patients often show high fusional reserves.
- Graves' ophthalmopathy. Exophthalmos and lid retraction are present.
- Intraorbital tumor. Proptosis may be present.
- Muscle entrapment. Usually, there is a history of trauma. Positive forced duction is present.
- Internuclear ophthalmoplegia. Adduction deficit. Fellow abducting eye demonstrates nystagmus. Brain stem disease or multiple sclerosis are possible.
- Myasthenia gravis. Often there is a confusing motility pattern. Often there is variable or alternating ptosis.

CRANIAL NERVE PALSIES

Third Nerve Palsy

- Characterized by ptosis with eye in the "down and out" position
- An isolated pupil-sparing palsy is most often ischemic vascular in origin.
- A blown pupil is often associated with an aneurysm.

Fourth Nerve Palsy

- Most often seen after trauma
- Cause sometimes never found
- Due to aneurysm or neoplasm in approximately 10% of cases

Sixth Nerve Palsy

- Diplopia is horizontal and worse when gaze is directed toward the involved eye.
- Esotropia is greater at distance than at near vision.

Workup

When more than one cranial nerve is involved, the source of the lesion is most often in the cavernous sinus. When the pupil is blown, angiography is indicated. The following tests are suggested for an isolated pupil-sparing cranial nerve palsy.

- Blood pressure
- Complete blood cell count
- Glucose tolerance test
- Sedimentation rate
- Venereal Disease Research Laboratory (VDRL) and fluorescent treponemal antibody absorption (FTA-ABS) tests
- Antinuclear antibody test
- Computed tomographic (CT) scan or, better, MRI of brain

Prognosis

If the cause is determined to be ischemic vascular (e.g., hypertension, diabetes), then recovery is expected within 90 days. The patient may choose to wear a patch to alleviate diplopia during the recovery period. The patient should be seen every 2–3 weeks, and the angle of strabismus should be remeasured on follow-up visits. The physician should rethink the diagnosis if multiple cranial nerves are involved, if the pupil is blown, if recovery does not occur, or if aberrant regeneration takes place.

NYSTAGMUS

There are multiple classification schemes for nystagmus, but the diagnosis and management can be simplified by determining a few basic features of the motility disturbance.

1. Is the motility disorder congenital (i.e., present within first few days after birth)?
2. Is the disorder conjugate (binocular) or dissociated (monocular or asymmetric)?
3. Is the nystagmus pendular (equal velocity in both directions) or jerk (possessing a fast and slow component)?
4. Is the nystagmus present in primary (straight ahead) gaze or only in eccentric gaze?

Congenital Nystagmus

Features

- Present at birth or during the perinatal period
- Horizontal in all gaze positions, although may have a rotary component in lateral gaze
- Bilateral and grossly symmetric in amplitude and frequency
- Disappears during sleep
- Patient does not experience oscillopsia (sensation of movement)

- Patient may assume a head position that minimizes the nystagmus (eyes in gaze position that minimizes the nystagmus—i.e., the null point).

Management

An eccentric gaze position (null point) or convergence may improve visual acuity by attenuating the nystagmus. Prism eyeglasses and surgery (muscle resection/recession) have variable efficacy.

Acquired Nystagmus

Binocular

Spasmus Nutans
Features:

- Onset at 4–14 months of age
- Generally horizontal, pendular nystagmus
- Rarely rotary or vertical
- Nystagmus may be unilateral, bilateral, or asymmetric.
- Associated with head nodding
- Occasionally associated with torticollis (abnormal head tilt)

Management:

- Radiologic imaging: CT scan or MRI to exclude intracranial mass
- Self-resolves in childhood

Latent Nystagmus
Features:

- Jerk nystagmus presents with occlusion of one eye.
- Fast component away from covered eye
- Good binocular visual acuity
- Decreased vision in nonoccluded eye due to nystagmus
- Can measure true monocular acuity by Polaroid glasses and vectographic slides or simply by placing high plus lens over fellow eye to blur but not disrupt binocularity

Table 10.2   Peripheral Versus Central Vestibular Disease

	Central	Peripheral
Vertigo severity	Mild	Severe
Auditory symptoms	Rare	Common
Character	Direction may change with gaze	Fast phase is constant
Inhibition with fixation	No	Yes

Primary-Position Jerk Nystagmus

A jerk nystagmus present with the patient gazing straight ahead in the primary position generally indicates a lesion of the vestibular apparatus. The lesion may be central or peripheral. The characteristics of the nystagmus may help differentiate a central lesion from a peripheral vestibular lesion (Table 10.2).

Features:

- Marked vertigo often indicates a peripheral lesion. Common etiologies are infectious disease, inflammation, or toxic agents.
- Visual fixation tends to inhibit nystagmus from peripheral vestibular disease.
- Lesions of the central vestibular apparatus usually are associated with mild vertigo, not inhibited by fixation.
- Common etiologies of central vestibular dysfunction include demyelinating disease, ischemia, and acoustic neuroma.

Specific Clinical Entities:

Wallenberg's Lateral Medullary Syndrome.   Wallenberg's lateral medullary syndrome is caused by occlusion of the posterior inferior cerebellar artery and consists of ipsilateral loss of facial pain and temperature sensation, contralateral loss in the trunk and limbs, Horner's syndrome, dysarthria, dysphagia, ipsilateral ataxia of the limbs, and nystagmus beating away from the lesion.

Periodic Alternating Nystagmus.   Typically if the patient is asked to hold his or her eyes in one position of gaze, cycles of jerk nystagmus appear in one direction, followed by no nystagmus or downbeating nystagmus, followed by nystagmus with the fast phase in the opposite direction. Periodic alternating nystagmus is caused by a lesion of the vestibular nucleus. Usually it is not associated with vertigo. Most patients should be investigated with MRI or other neuroimaging scans.

Upbeat Nystagmus.   Etiologies of upbeat nystagmus include drug-induced, cerebellar, and medullary lesions.

Downbeat Nystagmus.   Downbeat nystagmus usually indicates cervicomedullary disease. Common causes include Arnold-Chiari malformation, multiple sclerosis, stroke, communicating hydrocephalus, and drug intoxication.

Gaze-Evoked Nystagmus

Gaze-evoked nystagmus includes physiologic nystagmus (benign) as well as pathologic nystagmus (gaze paretic nystagmus).

- Physiologic or end-position nystagmus is an irregular nystagmus that is poorly sustained and occurs when the eyes are held in eccentric gaze. The fast component is toward the position of gaze.
- Gaze-paretic nystagmus is likewise seen in eccentric gaze but tends to be sustained and does not require the extreme eccentric gaze of end-point nystagmus. It may indicate a cerebellar lesion.
- Barbiturates, tranquilizers, and other drugs may also produce a gaze-evoked nystagmus. The nystagmus may be horizontal or vertical and may have a rotary component.
- A horizontal rotary nystagmus may be present in association with larger amplitude nystagmus in opposite gaze in patients with cerebellopontine angle lesions (e.g., acoustic neuromas).

Pendular Nystagmus

Horizontal nystagmus is characterized by slow pendular eye movements in primary gaze.

- May change to a jerk nystagmus in lateral gaze.
- Usually associated with sensory deprivation—i.e., reduced visual acuity. Etiologies include macular scarring, aniridia, albinism, and optic nerve hypoplasia.

See-Saw Nystagmus
"See-saw" nystagmus is characterized by torsional eye movements with one eye rising as the other falls.

• Associated with lesions of the third ventricle or upper brain stem

Convergence Retraction Nystagmus
The patient shows retraction of the globes with convergence-type eye movements in attempted upgaze.

• May be associated with dilated, unreactive pupils and papilledema
• Most commonly due to pineal gland tumor or midbrain lesion
• MRI is generally the preferred diagnostic imaging modality.

Dissociated Oscillations

Internuclear Ophthalmoplegia
Internuclear ophthalmoplegia (INO) is characterized by an adduction deficit in one eye with nystagmoid movement of the fellow abducting eye in attempted lateral gaze.

• Indicates a lesion of the medial longitudinal fasciculus.
• Vascular disease is the most common cause of unilateral internuclear ophthalmoplegia.
• Demyelinating disease (e.g., multiple sclerosis) is the most common cause of bilateral INO.
• Investigation of etiology generally includes MRI with specific attention to the brain stem.

Superior Oblique Myokymia
Small vertical and torsional eye movements are usually worse when gazing down and in.

• The patient may complain of "shaky" vision, blurred vision, or diplopia or offer only vague complaints.
• Most easily appreciated by the examiner with slit-lamp examination or during ophthalmoscopy
• Usually a benign condition that resolves spontaneously
• Consider carbamazepine for persistent, incapacitating cases.

Monocular Visual Deprivation (see Pendular Nystagmus above)

Spasmus Nutans (see discussion above)

Other Causes of Dissociated Oscillations

- Myasthenia gravis
- Cranial nerve paresis

OCULAR FLUTTER AND OPSOCLONUS

Ocular flutter and opsoclonus are eye movement abnormalities characterized by bursts of back-to-back saccades without an intersaccadic interval. Ocular flutter occurs only in the horizontal plane. Opsoclonus is chaotic and occurs in the vertical, torsional, and oblique planes.

Clinical Significance

- May occur as part of a postviral encephalopathy
- May represent a paraneoplastic effect of neuroblastoma in children
- May represent a paraneoplastic effect of visceral carcinoma in adults

NOTES

11

Visual Fields

Testing of the visual fields can be a useful tool for monitoring the progress of numerous ocular or neurologic disorders as well as uncovering the etiology of visual complaints (well defined or vague).

It is imperative that the clinician have a thorough understanding of ocular anatomy and the various conditions capable of producing visual field defects. Many instances of unnecessary "neurologic workups" and expensive radiologic studies can be cited as a result of misinterpretation of visual field test results.

The choice of visual field testing apparatus depends, in large part, on the type of field defect suspected and on the level of cooperation demonstrated by the patient. For instance, automated threshold perimetry of the central 30 degrees of visual field may be most appropriate for the glaucoma patient or for the patient suspected of having glaucoma. In the case of an elderly patient, however, the detail gained by this form of testing may be negated by inaccurate responses as a result of patient fatigue.

Functional vision loss may be confirmed by checking for tubular fields with the 1- and 2-m tangent screen. Subtle central visual field defects such as those found in tobacco-alcohol amblyopia can be missed with threshold tests; however, they may be easily demonstrated with a red Amsler grid on a black background.

In attempting to discover the etiology of vision loss in certain cases, it may be important to test the visual field of both eyes. Some patients, for instance, may mistakenly attribute a bilateral left field deficit as a vision loss in the left eye. A superior temporal field defect in an eye contralateral to an eye with unexplained visual acuity loss may direct the clinician to a chiasmal lesion.

IMPORTANT POINTS

1. Lesions located behind the optic chiasm produce visual field defects that respect the vertical meridian. One of the most common causes of bitemporal (or binasal) defects that cross the vertical meridian is bilaterally tilted optic discs.
2. Vascular etiologies (strokes) are more common causes of homonymous defects after age 40 years. Tumors are more common before age 40 years.
3. The borders of visual field defects created from vascular accidents tend to be steeper than the sloping borders found from intracranial tumors.
4. Associated clinical signs can be useful in localizing a lesion. Neurologic signs associated with retrochiasmal lesions follow.

OCCIPITAL LOBE

1. Internuclear ophthalmoplegia
2. Gaze palsies
3. Dysarthria (disturbance in articulation)
4. Dysphagia (difficulty swallowing)
5. Paresthesias (abnormal sensations such as tingling)
6. Drop attacks
7. Hemiparesis
8. Anton's syndrome (denial of blindness; seen in bilateral occipital lobe lesions)

PARIETAL LOBE

1. Asymmetric optokinetic nystagmus
2. Aphasia (inability to use words)
3. Alexia (inability to read)
4. Agraphia (inability to write)
5. Acalculia (inability to use numbers)
6. Prosopagnosia (inability to recognize familiar faces)
7. Palinopsia (images in blind half of field)

8. Spasticity of conjugate phase
9. Extinction (simultaneous presentation of targets necessary to demonstrate scotoma)
10. Corporal agnosia (unaware of body parts)
11. Right-left confusion
12. Apathy
13. Apraxia (inability to perform some movements)

TEMPORAL LOBE

1. Formed visual hallucinations
2. Déjà vu
3. Uncinate or psychomotor seizures
4. Olfactory hallucinations
5. Sensory aphasia
6. Hemiplegias
7. Alexia (loss of reading comprehension)
8. Agraphia (inability to write)
9. Transient conjugate deviation
10. Supranuclear facial weakness

BILATERAL FIELD DEFECTS

Commonly encountered bilateral and retrochiasmal field defects and their etiologies are shown in Fig. 11.1.

NOTES

Bilateral Central Scotomas

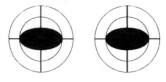

Bilateral Macular Disease
Bilateral Optic Neuritis
  (as in multiple sclerosis)
Tobacco-Alcohol Amblyopia
Nutritional Amblyopia
Hereditary Optic Neuropathy
  (e.g., Leber's)

Central Scotoma with Contralateral
Superior Quadrantanopia

Junctional Scotoma
  (chiasmal lesion with
  compression of optic
  nerve) (see etiologies
  below)

Bitemporal Hemianopias or
Superior Quadrantanopias

Pituitary Tumor
Meningioma
Craniopharyngioma
Gliomas
Aneurysm

Fig. 11.1   Bilateral field defects.

Superior Quadrantanopia

Temporal Lobe Lesion
  9:1 Tumor

Inferior Occipital Cortex
  4:1 Vascular Etiology

Inferior Quadrantanopia

Parietal Lobe Lesion
  1:1 Vascular vs. Tumor

Superior Occipital Cortex
  4:1 Vascular Etiology

Homonymous Hemianopia

No Localizing Value
Lesion may be located
anywhere along contralateral
retrochiasmal visual
pathway

Hemianopia with Macula Sparing

Occipital Lobe
  4:1 Vascular Etiology

12

Optic Nerve Abnormalities

PAPILLEDEMA VERSUS PSEUDOPAPILLEDEMA

The following ophthalmoscopic signs, when present, may be helpful in differentiating pseudopapilledema from true papilledema. The signs outlined below are believed to be most indicative of congenital disc elevation.

Pseudopapilledema Signs

- Absence of optic cup (optic cup usually retained in early papilledema)
- Abnormalities of the optic disc vasculature (e.g., trifurcations, loops, coils)
- Absence of peripapillary hemorrhages
- Optic nerve drusen

Table 12.1 describes common etiologies of the swollen optic disc.

PSEUDOTUMOR CEREBRI

Pseudotumor cerebri (benign intracranial hypertension) is an idiopathic increase in intracranial pressure presenting most commonly in women in the third decade of life. By definition, patients with pseudotumor cerebri must meet the following criteria:

1. Increased intracranial pressure on lumbar puncture
2. Normal head imaging scan
3. Normal cerebrospinal fluid composition

Table 12.1   The Swollen Disc: Common Etiologies and Their Differentiation

	Papilledema	Papillitis	Optic Neuropathy	Papillophlebitis
Laterality	Bilateral	Unilateral	Acutely unilateral	Unilateral
Vision loss	Transient (sec); usually normal acuity; enlarged blind spots	Usually central or cecocentral defects; red desaturation	Altitudinal loss most common	Usually good vision; may describe vague visual symptoms
Pupil	Normal	Marcus Gunn	Marcus Gunn	Normal
Other signs	Often headaches, nausea	Pain on eye movement	Tender scalp, appetite loss in giant cell	None
Commonly associated systemic disorders	Brain tumor; pseudotumor cerebri	Multiple sclerosis	Temporal arteritis; hypertension; diabetes	Often healthy young adults; occasionally in periarteritis and granulomatous vasculitis

Etiology

Although the most common condition associated with pseudotumor cerebri is obesity, a number of other conditions have been described as possible etiologies and should specifically be considered in making the diagnosis. Conditions associated with pseudotumor cerebri include:

- Obesity
- Pregnancy
- Vitamin A use
- Tetracycline use
- Nalidixic acid use
- Corticosteroid use or withdrawal
- Chronic obstructive pulmonary disease
- Middle ear disease
- Radical neck dissection
- Venous sinus thrombosis

Signs and Symptoms

- Papilledema
- Diplopia/esodeviations
- Headache (typically worse when prone in bed)
- Nausea and vomiting
- Transient obscurations of vision (lasting seconds and precipitated by changes in posture)
- Tinnitus
- Dizziness
- Enlarged blind spot on visual field testing
- More advanced disease can result in more severe vision loss and optic atrophy.

Management

Initial evaluation may include:

- Baseline evaluation including visual fields and color vision
- Blood pressure

- Evaluation of risk factors (e.g., medication use)
- Immediate magnetic resonance imaging (MRI) or computed tomography (CT) scan of the brain to rule out a mass
- Lumbar puncture including opening pressure
- Magnetic resonance venography (MRV) to rule out venous sinus thrombosis

Further management may include:

- Repeat examinations including visual fields and color vision, initially every 2–3 weeks
- Weight loss program if patient is obese
- Acetazolamide (Diamox) 250 mg PO qid. May increase to 500 mg PO qid.
- Optic nerve sheath decompression or lumbo-peritoneal shunts for resistant cases or when vision loss ensues

OPTIC NEURITIS

Optic neuritis means inflammation or demyelination of the optic nerve and should be differentiated from ischemic or compressive nerve injury as well as papilledema from increased intracranial pressure (see Table 12.1). Optic neuritis can be divided into three types based on the anatomic location of nerve involvement.

1. Papillitis: anterior swelling or inflammation can be identified with the ophthalmoscope.
2. Neuroretinitis: extension into the surrounding retina
3. Retrobulbar optic neuritis: the most common variant, in which the optic nerve involvement is too far posterior to be identified with the ophthalmoscope. The statement, "The patient sees nothing and the doctor sees nothing," is incorrect. The examiner should be able to identify a relative afferent pupillary defect (see the section on pupillary testing in Chap. 10).

Clinical Signs and Symptoms

- Sudden monocular decrease in visual acuity, which may progress over 2–5 days
- Often associated with retrobulbar pain, especially on movement
- Color vision loss/red desaturation (ask patient to compare brightness of colors between the two eyes using color plates or red cap of mydriatic eye drops)
- Visual field defect. Cecocentral defect is most common but may show arcuate or other defects as well.
- Afferent pupillary defect
- Most often affects women between 20 and 40 years of age

Management

- Most cases resolve with very good acuity. Monitor every 2–4 weeks.
- Suspicion of associated systemic conditions (viral infections [e.g., herpes zoster, mononucleosis, mumps, chickenpox], tuberculosis, syphilis, sarcoidosis) warrants laboratory testing and/or referral for complete blood cell count, rapid plasma reagin (RPR), fluorescent treponemal antibody absorption test (FTA-ABS), antinuclear antibody test, chest x-ray, etc.
- Atypical cases (chronic progressive course, bilateral cases, atypical age of patient, unusual associated features) may indicate the need for radiologic studies or consideration of another diagnosis (e.g., Leber's optic neuropathy, nutritional/toxic optic neuropathy, ischemic optic neuropathy, compressive lesions).
- Previous episodes or a history of other neurologic symptoms (e.g., paresthesias, diplopia) warrant an investigation for multiple sclerosis (e.g., MRI of brain).
- Serologic testing for anticardiolipin antibodies and cofactor may be indicated because this syndrome may mimic multiple sclerosis and result in optic neuritis.
- The Optic Neuritis Treatment Trial investigated the use of steroids in the treatment of optic neuritis when offered within 8 days of visual symptoms. The results suggest the following:

1. The use of high-dose IV steroids (250 mg methylprednisolone q6h) for 3 days followed by oral prednisone (1 mg/kg/day) for 11 days hastened visual recovery but provided no long-term benefit to vision.
2. This same treatment (high-dose IV steroids followed by oral steroids) seemed to provide temporary protection against new neurologic events consistent with multiple sclerosis, especially if demyelinating lesions were seen on MRI.
3. Oral steroids alone may be associated with an increased frequency of future attacks of optic neuritis and therefore should not be used.

ANTERIOR ISCHEMIC OPTIC NEUROPATHY

Anterior ischemic optic neuropathy (AION) is generally thought to be due to an infarction of the prelaminar optic nerve as a result of occlusion of the posterior ciliary arteries. Less commonly, infarction of the optic nerve posterior to the lamina cribrosa causes vision loss without oph-thalmoscopic signs. It is critical to differentiate AION due to giant cell arteritis from nonarteritic AION, because systemic steroids may prevent involvement of the fellow eye. Table 12.2 highlights the differences in clinical presentation between arteritic AION and nonarteritic AION.

Table 12.2   Arteritic Anterior Ischemic Optic Neuropathy (AION) Versus Nonarteritic AION

	Arteritic	*Nonarteritic*
Age	40–60	Over age 50
Associated physical symptoms	Headache, scalp tenderness, anorexia, weight loss, fever	Usually none
Other associated diseases	Temporal arteritis, polymyalgia rheumatica	Hypertension, diabetes, arterio-sclerosis
Sedimentation rate	Usually markedly elevated	Normal
Treatment	Steroids	No effective treatment

Signs and Symptoms

- Sudden, painless vision loss
- Usually a unilateral condition, although bilateral cases are not rare. Involvement of the fellow eye occurs frequently.
- Often an altitudinal visual field defect, but may be arcuate or any other pattern consistent with a prechiasmal lesion
- Afferent pupillary defect
- Pale swelling of the optic nerve head (diffuse or segmental)
- Often with peripapillary nerve fiber layer hemorrhages
- May be associated with cotton-wool spots or attenuated retinal vessels, or both
- Optic nerve atrophy commonly develops.
- Optic nerve cupping similar to that seen in glaucoma is not unusual.
- The pseudo–Foster Kennedy syndrome refers to optic nerve atrophy due to a remote AION as well as pale swelling of the optic nerve in the fellow eye due to recent AION. This mimics the ophthalmoscopic appearance of a chiasmal mass.

Management

- History and physical examination with search for symptoms of giant cell arteritis—i.e., temporal headache, pain on chewing, low-grade fever, anorexia, weight loss
- Blood tests: complete blood cell count with differential and stat sedimentation rate. Note that it is possible to have arteritic AION with a normal sedimentation rate.
- CT scan or MRI only for atypical cases
- Start immediately on high-dose steroids (e.g., prednisone 100 mg/day PO or methylprednisone 250 mg IV q6h for one or two doses before switching to oral steroids) if arteritic AION is suspected based on age, erythrocyte sedimentation rate, or associated symptoms. Consider starting patient concomitantly on antiulcer medications.
- Confirm giant cell arteritis with temporal artery biopsy within 1 week of starting steroids.

- After 2–4 weeks the steroid dose is usually tapered using erythrocyte sedimentation rates as a guide.
- There is some evidence that daily use of aspirin decreases the incidence of nonarteritic AION in the fellow eye (although the benefit may not hold up long term). Many clinicians prescribe one aspirin daily for prophylaxis.

OPTIC NERVE GLIOMA

Optic nerve gliomas are the most common optic nerve tumors. They are usually composed of low-grade astrocytes, although rarely, a malignant chiasmal glioma occurs. The tumor tends to occur in childhood and adolescence. There is a higher incidence in neurofibromatosis. Bilateral cases suggest neurofibromatosis.

Signs and Symptoms

- Painless vision loss
- Proptosis
- Optic nerve atrophy
- Afferent pupillary defect
- Gliosis of the optic nervehead
- Chiasmal involvement may produce variable vision defects without proptosis.

Management

- CT is generally preferred for orbital involvement. MRI is best for chiasmal or hypothalamic involvement.
- For tumors affecting a single optic nerve, sparing the chiasm and producing proptosis and vision loss, the treatment is transcranial excision of the nerve from the globe to the chiasm.
- For chiasmal tumors, malignant tumors, and multicentric tumors, the usual treatment is radiation therapy.

OPTIC NERVE SHEATH MENINGIOMA

Optic nerve sheath meningiomas are the second most common optic nerve tumor after gliomas. They are benign neoplasms and tend to affect middle-aged adults.

Signs and Symptoms

- Gradually progressive vision loss
- Chronic optic disc swelling
- Optic atrophy
- Optociliary shunt vessels
- Proptosis
- Orbital pain or headache in 50% of patients

Management

- CT scan: Diffuse tubular enlargement is very common. Frequently the meningioma is calcified.
- Surgery is usually reserved only for those patients with blindness, severe proptosis, or extension toward the optic canal.

NOTES

13

Glaucoma

Glaucoma is a disease that affects up to 2% of the population over the age of 40 years. In addition, a certain number of younger patients are affected. The notion that glaucoma is a disease that results from high intraocular pressures (IOPs) has been challenged by the observation that a number of patients develop or continue to lose vision in spite of "normal" IOP. It is probably best to consider glaucoma as an optic neuropathy of multifactorial etiology. High IOP is a risk factor and indeed the only factor that is modified by standard glaucoma therapy. In the future it is expected that neuroprotective or neurorescue agents will play a role in glaucoma management. The investigation and monitoring of glaucoma primarily involves evaluation of the following three characteristics:

- Level of IOP
- Amount of optic atrophy (cupping) or nerve fiber loss
- Change in visual field function or loss of visual field

Glaucoma may be a primary condition, perhaps with heredity playing a role, or secondary to another disorder such as neovascularization or damage to the angle from blunt trauma.

PRIMARY OPEN-ANGLE GLAUCOMA

In primary open-angle glaucoma (POAG), the angle appears open at all times. No obvious obstruction to outflow is apparent clinically, and there are no associated ocular diseases. This is by far the most common type of glaucoma.

Diagnosis

Most patients suspected of having POAG present with increased or asymmetric cupping or high IOPs. Some patients present with vision loss characteristic of advanced glaucoma.

The investigation of suspected glaucoma still consists mainly of IOP measurements, an optic nervehead evaluation, and an assessment of the visual fields. Other factors may have a role in the decision as to whether it is advisable to initiate therapy, and newer diagnostic procedures provide useful additive information, but these three time-honored tests remain the cornerstone of glaucoma investigation.

- IOP measurement: Applanation tonometry, because of its reproducibility and accuracy, is indicated whenever possible in the evaluation of glaucoma. Multiple measurements are often advisable. It is recognized that normal diurnal variations and the exaggerated IOP fluctuations often found in glaucoma patients may limit the usefulness of a single pressure measurement. In addition, there are a group of glaucoma patients with "normal" IOPs.
- Optic nerve evaluation: The optic nerveheads should be examined stereoscopically using an indirect condensing lens and a slit-lamp. The average cup-to-disc ratio (C/D) in whites is approximately .25. In blacks it is approximately .35. Large variations in cup size exist among the general population. While such clinical findings as notching and vertical elongation of the cup are helpful diagnostic signs, many patients show only a generalized enlargement of the cup. This may make it impossible to determine whether a cup is glaucomatous or simply physiologically enlarged. Stereoscopic photographs may be useful to determine whether cupping is progressive. An isolated disc hemorrhage (Drance hemorrhage) is a fairly reliable indicator of glaucomatous optic atrophy and a predictor of future visual field loss.
- Visual fields: Visual field defects occur relatively late in the course of the disease. Automated perimeters using threshold strategies are the most reliable in picking up glaucomatous defects. They are

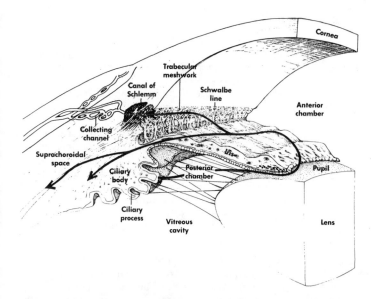

Fig. 13.1 Pathway of aqueous humor flow. Abnormalities of the anterior chamber angle may be visible with the use of gonioscopy. (Reprinted with permission from F Newell. Ophthalmology: Principles and Concepts [7th ed]. St. Louis: Mosby-Year Book, 1992.)

also useful in monitoring progression. Visual fields should be repeated every 6–12 months.

- Gonioscopy: Many clinicians perform gonioscopy on all patients with glaucoma and those suspected of having glaucoma. Other clinicians reserve this procedure for patients who are suspected of having a secondary glaucoma, who are unresponsive to initial therapy, or who appear to have a narrow angle by slit-lamp estimation (Fig. 13.1).

Pitfalls in Diagnosis

- Great variability exists in the level of IOP tolerated by patients. There is no "magic number." Some patients have severe glaucoma at an IOP of 17 or lower. Other patients can tolerate an IOP of 29 and greater for many years with no apparent loss of visual function.
- Individual variations in the size of the optic cup may make it impossible to differentiate between normal physiologic cupping and glaucomatous atrophy.
- Visual field loss is a rather late indicator of glaucomatous atrophy. Up to 60% of axons can be lost without a localized visual field defect.
- Glaucoma can have numerous etiologies and contributing factors. In fact, glaucoma may not be a single disease but a group of disorders. It may be, for instance, that glaucomatous atrophy from open-angle glaucoma has a completely different etiology than that found in progressive low-tension glaucoma.

Initiation of Therapy

Numerous new diagnostic tests and approaches are put forth every year, all in an effort to separate those patients who need pressure-lowering therapy from those who do not. There is often disagreement as to when to initiate therapy. Many clinicians will not wait for an unequivocal visual field defect and documented progression of cupping before initiating therapy. Patients with both of these findings require therapy to lower IOP, regardless of the level of IOP.

The following guidelines are offered to the clinician who is unfamiliar with glaucoma management. Most clinicians will eventually develop their own procedure. It is recognized that there are numerous factors, such as concerns of patient compliance and patient apprehension, to cause one to deviate from these guidelines.

Initiate Therapy

- IOP consistently >28
- IOP 22–28: C/D asymmetry, glaucomatous cupping, notching, nerve fiber layer dropout, or condition associated with glaucoma

(e.g., pigmentary dispersion, pseudoexfoliation, young patients with a strong family history of glaucoma)
- IOP <22: Glaucomatous cupping, visual field defects (be sure to rule out other causes)

Monitor

- IOP 22–28: Healthy nerveheads, no field defects, uncomplicated reliable patient
- IOP <22: Suspicious cups, no field defects

Goals of Therapy

The goal of therapy is obviously to prevent initial or further vision loss. This is accomplished by lowering the IOP. Therapy is usually medical initially. Argon laser trabeculoplasty (ALT), filtering procedures, or other procedures are options if IOP cannot be lowered to a sufficient level medically.

Unfortunately, there is no way to be certain of what level of IOP is safe for a particular patient. Therefore, patients need to be monitored for progression of cupping or visual field loss.

It is well known that eyes that have suffered marked optic atrophy seem prone to further damage at lower pressures than eyes with little or no glaucomatous atrophy. Eyes with severe damage therefore need to be treated more aggressively not only because of the amount of visual loss already incurred but also because a lower pressure is probably necessary to halt the glaucomatous process. An eye with advanced cupping and visual field loss may need to have the pressure reduced to 10 or 11 to prevent further vision compromise. On the other hand, the clinician may be content with an IOP of 20 for an eye with only early damage. One should never be content just looking at the numbers. Periodic reevaluations are a must.

Therapy Guidelines

- Choose the agent most likely to work with the lowest chance of adverse effects and the greatest likelihood of being used. Beta blockers and pilocarpine are the most common first-line agents. A beta blocker, however, would be a poor choice for a patient with marked asthma. Newer agents such as prostaglandins, alpha-adrenergic agents, and topical anhydrase inhibitors are increasingly being used as first- or second-line agents. Pilocarpine's side effects have caused this agent to fall out of favor, but select patients can tolerate this medication with good therapeutic results. See Table 22.8 for common agents used in glaucoma management.

- Start with lower dosages; one agent at a time.
- Evaluate response soon (1–2 weeks).
- Make sure the patient has used the drop before reevaluation. Record the time the medication was last used.
- If first medication shows no effect, discontinue and try another rather than adding.
- When adding medications, use those most likely to be additive in effect.
- Forewarn of potential side effects.
- Explain how to administer medication and when.
- Question the patient on follow-up as to how he or she is using medication.
- Make sure the patient understands the purpose of the medication— i.e., to prevent visual loss rather than improve vision or comfort.

Effect of Systemic Medications

Numerous systemic medications have been found to have an effect on glaucoma. Patients and their physicians will often ask, "Is it safe to use this drug?" In most cases the answer should be "maybe."

Not all glaucoma patients will lose control of their IOP because they have started a medication with a warning about glaucoma. For instance, certain over-the-counter cold remedies will advise against their use for glaucoma patients. These medications may raise IOP through pupil dilation and compromise the anterior chamber angle. This may mean very little to a patient already on a miotic drug or with very wide open angles. If it is decided that there is a significant benefit to the use of a certain drug, ask to see the patient shortly after it is started to check IOP. Adjust glaucoma medications or the systemic drug as appropriate to maintain control.

One antihistamine said to have no effect on glaucoma is astemizole (Hismanal).

JUVENILE OPEN-ANGLE GLAUCOMA

Occasionally glaucoma that is not associated with clinically recognizable angle abnormality develops in children. There is often a family history of glaucoma. Medical therapy should be attempted first, but surgery is often necessary.

LOW-TENSION GLAUCOMA

Symptoms of low-tension glaucoma include progressive cupping and loss of visual field despite normal IOPs. This condition needs to be differentiated from "burnt out" glaucoma and other conditions simulating glaucoma (such as ischemic optic neuropathy). Diurnal IOP measurements can be helpful in documenting maximal pressures. Efforts to associate low tension with systemic hypotension have been less than impressive. Treatment, as in POAG, involves lowering IOP. Determining a safe level of IOP can be challenging. Surgery may be necessary.

PIGMENTARY GLAUCOMA

Pigmentary glaucoma is associated with pigmentary dispersion syndrome and is characterized by deposition of pigment on the back of the cornea (Krukenberg's spindle), trabecular meshwork, and other intraocular structures. Loss of pigment may result in transillumination defects involving the midperipheral iris. The IOP in pigmentary glaucoma tends to be prone to large fluctuations and can increase with exercise or pupillary dilation. Ultrasound studies show that the iris chafing may be due to posterior bowing of the iris. Laser iridotomy may reverse the iris bowing but has not been proved to produce clinical benefit.

Management

- Workup is the same as for POAG (see above).
- Pilocarpine is the preferred first-line agent because it limits iris movement and contact with the lens zonules, which are believed to be the source of pigment dispersion, but it is poorly tolerated by most young patients.
- This glaucoma tends to respond well to laser trabeculoplasty.
- Consider laser iridotomy to correct posterior iris bowing.

PSEUDOEXFOLIATIVE GLAUCOMA

Glaucoma associated with the pseudoexfoliative syndrome is characterized by the presence of dandruff-like flakes or a gray membrane with curled edges on the anterior surface of the lens. The material may be responsible for outflow obstruction. Treatment is the same as for open-angle glaucoma. This glaucoma also responds well to laser trabeculoplasty.

TRAUMATIC (CONTUSION) GLAUCOMA

Traumatic (contusion) glaucoma is characterized by elevated IOP after trauma to the eye. Glaucoma may develop shortly after injury or years later. Elevated pressures may occur as a result of disruption of angle structures, and an angle recess may be seen on gonioscopy. Treatment is the same as for POAG although these eyes show varied responses to topical medications. They usually do not respond well to laser trabeculoplasty, and filtering procedures are commonly required to bring IOPs to an acceptable level.

UVEITIC GLAUCOMA

Ocular hypotony has classically been thought to be a part of uveitis, but on occasion, presumably as a result of infiltration of the trabecular meshwork by inflammatory cells, secondary glaucoma may develop. In addition, synechia formation can act to elevate IOP. It is important to differentiate glaucoma caused by intraocular inflammation from narrow-angle glaucoma, which may produce intraocular inflammation. The following are uveitic conditions that may lead to secondary glaucoma:

- Acute iritis or iridocyclitis
- Recurrent and chronic iritis
- Surgically induced uveitis (retained cortex or inflammation associated with iris fixated or anterior chamber intraocular lens)
- Phacolytic glaucoma (associated with hypermature cataract)
- Glaucomatocyclitic crisis (Posner-Schlossman syndrome): characterized by attacks of elevated IOP lasting 1–3 weeks and associated with epithelial edema and low-grade iritis. The eye appears relatively uninflamed.
- Heterochromatic cyclitis: low-grade cyclitis with iris atrophy, abnormal transillumination, and lightening of iris color

Management

- Workup to determine the etiology when unknown. See Chapter 6 on uveitis.
- Treatment of uveitis with steroids as appropriate. Steroids are not effective in Fuchs' heterochromatic cyclitis.
- Cycloplegics may be indicated.
- Beta blockers or other aqueous suppressants are usually first-line agents.
- Keep in mind that steroids can secondarily increase IOP. Consider this in patients who initially respond well but later are difficult to control.
- Uveitis secondary to a hypermature lens requires surgical management.
- Uveitis secondary to retained crystalline lens material after cataract surgery can often be managed medically. Large fragments may require surgical removal.
- Replacement or removal of the intraocular lens may be required in pseudophakic uveitis.
- Always consider the possibility of infectious endophthalmitis in cases of uveitis appearing after intraocular surgery.

- Laser or surgical iridectomies may be necessary in cases of posterior synechiae and iris bombé.
- Recalcitrant cases of glaucoma associated with uveitis may require filter procedures with antimetabolites or setons.

NEOVASCULAR GLAUCOMA

Elevated IOP develops as a result of fibrovascular membrane growth over the trabecular meshwork. Neovascularization develops primarily as a result of retinal or anterior segment ischemia or inflammation. Of utmost importance is the identification of the predisposing pathologic condition.

Signs and Symptoms

- Painful red eye. Patient will usually report that the involved eye previously had poor vision.
- Tufts of irregular vessels on iris surface or trabecular meshwork
- Peripheral anterior synechiae may lead to narrow or occluded angles. Examine the angle of the fellow eye to differentiate from primary narrow-angle glaucoma.
- High IOP may lead to corneal edema. Reduction of IOP and topical hyperosmotics (e.g., glycerin) may be required for adequate visualization.
- Often may present with an associated anterior uveitis

Management

Reduction of Intraocular Pressures Medically

- Topical beta blockers
- Carbonic anhydrase inhibitors (acetazolamide or Neptazane)
- Oral isosorbide or glycerol. Remember that glycerol should be avoided in diabetic patients.
- Avoid miotic drugs.
- Topical atropine and steroids to reduce inflammation

Identification of Etiology

See below for etiologies of rubeosis iridis. When the etiology is unclear because of cloudy media:

- Examine fellow eye for evidence of diabetic retinopathy.
- Auscultate carotids. Search for history of stroke or transient ischemic attacks.
- Consider noninvasive carotid studies (e.g., duplex scan).
- B scan ultrasound of orbit to rule out retinal detachment or intraocular tumor
- Erythrocyte sedimentation rate to screen for giant cell arteritis; temporal artery biopsy if suspicion is high

Common Causes of Rubeosis Iridis

- Diabetic retinopathy
- Central retinal vein occlusion
- Central retinal artery occlusion
- Branch retinal vein occlusion
- Carotid occlusive disease
- Chronic retinal detachment
- Sickle cell retinopathy
- Retinopathy of prematurity
- Eale's disease
- Giant cell arteritis
- Aortic arch syndrome
- Chronic uveitis
- Uveal melanoma

Definitive Surgical Management

- Panretinal photocoagulation if media allows for retinal ischemia
- For cloudy media, transcleral panretinal cryotherapy, vitrectomy with panretinal endolaser photocoagulation, and/or cyclodestructive treatment may be necessary.
- Goniophotocoagulation may delay or prevent angle closure.

- Conventional filtration surgery can be performed in a quiet eye that maintains useful vision after vessel regression. Antimetabolites or setons may be necessary.
- Alcohol block or enucleation may be necessary for a painful eye without useful vision.

PHACOLYTIC GLAUCOMA

A rapid rise in IOP may be associated with a hypermature cataract that leaks protein through an intact lens capsule. The etiology is believed to be obstruction of the meshwork with macrophages and lens debris. Medical treatment is ineffective, making surgical removal of the lens a necessity.

PHACOANAPHYLACTIC GLAUCOMA

Phacoanaphylactic glaucoma is very rare. It is an immunologic response to lens protein and occurs after trauma or surgery. It is associated with a violated lens capsule and requires previous sensitization. Treatment is removal of the lens.

ESSENTIAL IRIS ATROPHY

Essential iris atrophy is characterized by a patchy loss of iris stroma and distortion or displacement of the pupil. Usually it is a unilateral condition, and signs become noticeable in early or middle adult life. Synechia of the iris to the cornea may develop, thus obstructing outflow. Some patients show a corneal endothelial dystrophy and edema. This group of patients is classified separately as Chandler's syndrome. Treatment is the same as for POAG. Hypertonic saline (5% sodium chloride) may be indicated if corneal edema is present.

PRIMARY INFANTILE (CONGENITAL) GLAUCOMA

Congenital glaucoma occurs within the first 3 years of life. Eighty percent of cases manifest within the first year of life. Males are slightly more affected. Increased distensibility of the globe is responsible for many of the characteristic findings not seen in the adult glaucomas. Another unique feature is the reversal of cupping that can occur once pressure is brought under control.

Signs and Symptoms

- Photophobia, epiphora, and blepharospasm
- Buphthalmos (globe enlargement): Horizontal corneal diameters greater than 11 mm in term infants and greater than 12 mm in 1-year-old infants are suspicious.
- Corneal edema
- Haab's striae (horizontal breaks in Descemet's membrane)
- Axial enlargement and resultant myopia
- Optic cup enlargement
- IOP greater than 20 mm Hg

Management

Measurement of IOP can sometimes be accomplished in the office while the infant bottle-feeds. Many children require examination under anesthesia, but keep in mind that general anesthesia can dramatically lower IOP. In some children, examination in the operating room can be accomplished under short-term sedation with oral midazolam (Versed) or with ketamine, neither of which lower IOP.

- In the newborn with glaucoma, rubella and Lowe's syndrome (aminoaciduria) should be ruled out. In an otherwise healthy child, no systemic evaluation is necessary.
- Medical management is typically only short term until definitive surgical treatment can be offered. Topical carbonic anhydrase inhibitors, alpha-adrenergic agents, prostaglandins, and beta blockers have all been used.
- Goniotomy or trabeculotomy are typically the procedures of choice. Individual cases may require filtering procedures or aqueous drainage devices.

Other Conditions Associated with Glaucoma

Congenital abnormalities can result in glaucoma at birth or later. These abnormalities are often evident clinically.

1. Aniridia: 50–75% of cases are associated with glaucoma.
2. Sturge-Weber syndrome: characterized by the presence of a facial cutaneous hemangioma (port-wine stain). Glaucoma commonly occurs in infancy but may occur at a later age. Increased episcleral venous pressure is the most likely reason for glaucoma in these patients.
3. Neurofibromatosis (von Recklinghausen's disease): Glaucoma is associated with 50% of cases with a plexiform neurofibroma of the upper lid.
4. Persistent hyperplastic primary vitreous is associated with angle-closure glaucoma.
5. Lowe's (oculocerebrorenal) syndrome is an X-linked disorder associated with cataracts and glaucoma. It is also associated with failure to thrive, mental retardation, and aminoaciduria.
6. Iridocorneal dysgenesis, characterized by:
   a. Embryotoxin: prominent Schwalbe's line
   b. Axenfeld's anomaly: embryotoxin with attached iris strands (50% incidence of glaucoma)
   c. Reiger's anomaly: embryotoxin, iris strands, and hypoplasia of iris stroma (60% incidence of glaucoma)
   d. Posterior keratoconus: posterior corneal depression
   e. Iridogoniodysgenesis: iris strands to Schwalbe's line, hypoplasia of anterior iris stroma
   f. Peter's anomaly: posterior corneal defect and leukoma. May be associated with abnormalities of the anterior chamber angle.
   g. Anterior chamber cleavage syndrome: combination of central and peripheral anterior chamber cleavage abnormalities

ACUTE ANGLE-CLOSURE GLAUCOMA

Acute angle-closure glaucoma is characterized by closure of the angle with a sudden increase in IOP. It should be distinguished from malignant glaucoma. In addition to markedly elevated IOP, the following conditions may also be present:

Signs and Symptoms

- Shallow angle in fellow eye
- Mid-dilated pupil
- Steamy cornea (corneal edema)
- Cells in anterior chamber
- Glaukomflecken (small white spots beneath the anterior lens capsule in the pupillary zone)
- Stromal atrophy of the iris
- Pain, lacrimation, nausea

Management

The mainstay of therapy for the patient with narrow-angle glaucoma is peripheral iridectomy. This is most commonly accomplished with a yttrium aluminum garnet (YAG) or argon laser. In the case of an acute narrow-angle glaucoma attack, it may be necessary to break the attack medically before proceeding with iridectomy.

The following medications should be administered, keeping in mind the patient's health status and medical condition at the time of presentation:

- Intravenous acetazolamide, or parenteral mannitol, and/or oral glycerin (nausea may prevent successful administration of oral agents)
- Topical beta blocker (timolol or other)
- Topical 1% or 2% pilocarpine administered every 10 minutes

Once the attack is successfully reversed, the patient should be kept on miotic drugs until iridectomy can be performed. As a general rule, the fellow eye should also be kept on miotics and an iridectomy performed in it if the angle is felt to be occludable.

CHRONIC ANGLE-CLOSURE GLAUCOMA

Chronic angle-closure glaucoma is characterized by small, intermittent attacks of elevated pressure and closure of the angle. The angle may not close around the entire circumference. Patients with this condition may not have symptoms and may present as would a patient with POAG. Gonioscopy and diurnal IOPs can aid in the differential diagnosis. As in acute angle-closure glaucoma, peripheral iridotomies are a mainstay of treatment.

MALIGNANT GLAUCOMA

Malignant glaucoma occurs most commonly in patients who have had intraocular surgery or laser treatment. Aqueous is misdirected into the vitreous, which forces the lens-iris diaphragm anteriorly and causes shallowing and eventual closure of the angle. Unlike acute narrow-angle glaucoma, the fellow eye typically demonstrates a normal or wide open chamber angle. Also, peripheral iridectomies are not curative. Miotics may worsen the block.

Signs and Symptoms

- Shallow peripheral and central anterior chamber
- Often follows intraocular surgery including filter procedures or laser peripheral iridotomies
- High IOP
- Patent iridotomy

Management

- Cycloplegic agents
- Topical and/or systemic antiglaucoma medications (not miotic drugs)
- Mannitol 12.5–25.0 g IV
- The definitive treatment involves rupture of the anterior hyaloid face with a YAG laser or, in intractable cases, vitreous surgery.

NOTES

14

Retinal Abnormalities

FLUORESCEIN ANGIOGRAPHY

Fluorescein angiography is a technique to study retinal and choroidal circulation. Fluorescein dye is injected intravenously. Retinal photographs are taken as the dye circulates in the retinal and choroidal vasculature. The retinal vessels have tight junctions and do not leak fluorescein. The choroidal vessels are porous, but leakage beneath or into the sensory retina is prevented by the retinal pigmented epithelium (RPE). Abnormalities seen in fluorescein angiography include hypofluorescence and hyperfluorescence.

Causes of Hypofluorescence

- Blockage by blood or pigment
- Nonperfusion of vessels: choroidal or retinal

Causes of Hyperfluorescence

- Leakage from retinal vessels
- Leakage from the choroid through a defect in the retinal pigmented epithelium
- Pooling into a fluid space
- Window defects. RPE cells that lack pigment allow transmission (not leakage) of fluorescence from the underlying choroid.

Leakage   Gradual marked increase in fluorescence with increasingly blurred borders

Staining	Gradual increase in fluorescence with more distinct borders
Pooling	Accumulation of fluorescein with distinct borders
Window defects	Early hyperfluorescence with gradual fade

ACUTE RETINAL NECROSIS

Acute retinal necrosis is a peripheral necrotizing retinitis thought to be caused by herpes zoster, herpes simplex 1 or 2, or cytomegalovirus. It is unclear why only some individuals infected with these viruses manifest the retinitis. It is also unknown why infection with each of these different viruses can present the same clinical picture. The condition may be unilateral or bilateral. The patient may or may not give a history of preceding mucocutaneous infection.

Signs and Symptoms

- Confluent peripheral necrotizing retinitis
- Arteritis
- Vitreitis
- Anterior uveitis
- Episcleritis
- Ocular hypertension
- May progress to optic nerve involvement or retinal detachment, or both

Management

- Uveitis and ocular hypertension may be treated with topical prednisolone, cycloplegic agents (e.g., homatropine), and beta blockers (e.g., timolol, betaxolol).
- Treat immunocompetent retinitis with systemic acyclovir—i.e., 10.0–12.5 mg/kg IV (adjusted for renal status) qd in three divided doses for at least 7 days then PO acyclovir 800 mg five times daily for 1 month (depending on severity and immune status). Patients with acquired immune deficiency disorder may be treated with IV

ganciclovir or foscarnet and/or IV acyclovir 20 mg/kg (adjusted for renal status) in three divided doses.
- Aspirin 650 mg/day for 1–2 months for arteritis and optic disc swelling
- Prednisone 40–80 mg/day PO *after* 1 or 2 days of acyclovir treatment. Continue for 1 week with gradual tapering for at least another 3–4 weeks.
- Consider a triple row of laser photocoagulation to posterior extent of retinal lesions for prophylaxis of retinal detachment.

PROGRESSIVE OUTER RETINAL NECROSIS

Progressive outer retinal necrosis is a necrotizing retinitis involving deeper retinal layers seen in patients with acquired immune deficiency syndrome (AIDS). Like acute retinal necrosis, it is believed to be secondary to the herpes zoster virus. Patients show evidence of a multifocal deep retinitis with minimal vitreitis. The retinal vasculature is relatively spared. Two-thirds of patients have had a cutaneous zoster infection. The disease tends to progress very rapidly, with coalescence of lesions, eventual full-thickness involvement, and a high retinal detachment rate.

Management

Triple treatment consists of acyclovir (20 mg/kg IV qd in three divided doses), IV induction with ganciclovir or foscarnet, and intravitreal injections of foscarnet 2,400 µg in 0.1 ml three times weekly.

CYSTOID MACULAR EDEMA

Accumulation of fluid from parafoveal capillaries creates macular edema in a discrete cystic, flower-petal arrangement. The fluid may appear yellow but is often clear and cannot be seen by direct ophthalmoscopy.

A fundus contact lens, 60 D or 90 D indirect lens, or fluorescein angiography is often necessary for detection. The edema is most often seen in association with:

- Cataract surgery
- Retinal vein occlusions
- Uveitis
- Retinitis pigmentosa
- Diabetic retinopathy
- Epinephrine therapy in aphakes/pseudophakes

Treatment

- Treat underlying disorder.
- Consider laser photocoagulation for edema associated with retinal vein occlusion or diabetic retinopathy.
- Lysis of incarcerated vitreous wick in aphakes/pseudophakes
- Topical, subtenous, and/or oral steroids in uveitis, postsurgically
- Carbonic anhydrase inhibitors
- Topical nonsteroidal anti-inflammatory drugs (e.g., ketorolac trimethamine 0.5% drops four times daily)
- Oral nonsteroidal anti-inflammatory drugs (e.g., ibuprofen)
- Hyperbaric oxygen

MACULAR HOLE

Macular holes are defects of the sensory retina centered over the fovea. They may be caused by vitreous traction on the retina or progression from a macular cyst. It is important to differentiate macular holes from conditions that may simulate them, such as chorioretinal atrophy, macular degeneration, and pseudoholes (holes in epiretinal membranes overlying the macula). Examination with a fundus contact lens or indirect condensing lens with a slit-lamp should be performed.

Stages

Stage I: Yellow spot or ring in center of the fovea with loss of foveal reflex/depression

Stage II: Full-thickness retinal dehiscence
Stage III: Overt macular hole

Signs and Symptoms

- Decreased visual acuity (often 20/200 or worse)
- Central scotoma on Amsler grid testing
- Appears as a depressed red circular lesion often with small yellow tags of tissue in the base of the hole
- A gray surrounding ring of subretinal fluid is common.
- Patients should describe a "break" in the line of a slit-lamp beam if a thin beam is projected directly through the lesion (positive Watzke-Allen test). A macular cyst may not have a full break.

Management

- Rarely progresses to retinal detachment. This requires surgery if it occurs.
- There is no effective treatment for the actual hole, but surgery can be effective in inducing resolution of the cuff of subretinal fluid, thus decreasing the size of the scotoma and improving vision.
- Vitrectomy to separate the posterior hyaloid from the inner retinal surface may have a role in the treatment of stage I also.

CENTRAL SEROUS CHOROIDOPATHY

- Localized macular detachment with symptoms of metamorphopsia and mild to moderate visual acuity loss
- Visual acuity is usually 20/20 to 20/80.
- Most commonly affects men aged 20–50 years
- May be induced by systemic corticosteroid therapy
- Contact fundus lens or 20 D, 60 D, or 90 D condensing lens usually required to detect elevation of sensory retina
- Must differentiate from sensory/retinal pigment epithelium detachment associated with age-related macular degeneration. The wet

form of macular degeneration is more common in older patients
and is associated with drusen and murky fluid/hemorrhage.

Management

- Complete eye examination, including dilation and Amsler grid testing
- Fluorescein angiography for persistent cases, if needed for differential diagnosis or before photocoagulation
- Monitor monthly. Consider laser photocoagulation for cases that
fail to resolve in 4–6 months.

EPIRETINAL MEMBRANE

Epiretinal membrane is also known as preretinal membrane, cello-
phane maculopathy, macular pucker, and surface wrinkling maculopathy. The membrane is caused by the growth and contraction of a
translucent membrane growing on the surface of the retina (usually
in the macular region). It is seen after retinal vein occlusion, retinal
detachment, intraocular surgery, trauma, posterior vitreous detachment, or uveitis, or it may be idiopathic in nature.

Clinical Signs

- May appear as a glistening sheen on surface of the retina, often
with fine wrinkles and folds
- May progress to a thick gray-white membrane with contraction,
causing gross distortion of retina
- Decreased vision
- Metamorphopsia
- May mimic appearance of macular hole

Treatment

- The only treatment is surgical—i.e., peeling of the membrane, which
is generally not attempted until vision deteriorates to 20/60 or lower.

POSTERIOR VITREOUS DETACHMENT

Posterior vitreous detachment is caused by a condensation and subsequent collapse of the vitreous humor and peeling away of the posterior vitreal surface from the surface of the retina. The main concern is that in areas where the vitreous is firmly adherent to the retina, such as around the border of lattice degeneration, vitreal collapse may result in a retinal tear and predispose to retinal detachment.

Clinical Signs and Symptoms

- The patient may describe flashing lights that last for a few seconds (versus minutes often with zig-zag pattern in migraine). These lights indicate vitreal traction.
- New floaters. May appear as a cobweb, ring, blob, etc.
- May be completely asymptomatic
- May produce hemorrhage on optic nerve, on retinal surface, or in vitreous as a result of traction over a retinal vessel
- The examiner may note a veil-like curtain, which is the posterior surface of the vitreous humor, with a fundus contact lens, 60 D or 90 D condensing lens, or slit-lamp behind the crystalline lens and in front of the retina.
- A "smoke ring" floater may appear suspended over the posterior pole.

Management

- Dilated fundus examination with binocular, indirect ophthalmoscopy to rule out a retinal break
- If no breaks are found, educate the patient about the symptoms of a retinal tear or detachment (e.g., curtain appearing over vision, new onset of "pepper-like" floaters). Instruct the patient to seek prompt attention if these are noted.
- Reexamine fresh vitreal detachments without breaks in 6 weeks.
- Table 14.1 describes common peripheral retina disorders.

Table 14.1   Peripheral Retinal Disorders

Disorder	Clinical Characteristics	Management
Lattice degeneration	Cigar-shaped lesions oriented parallel to ora; may have associated atrophic holes; if retinal vessels pass through, sclerosis gives lattice appearance; vitreous condensation at borders	Consider prophylactic treatment in fellow eye of retinal detachment, aphakes or patients in whom cataract surgery is planned; atrophic holes are not an indication for treatment
Atrophic retinal holes	Small circular area of missing sensory retina gives brighter burgundy appearance; may have surrounding cuff of edema; *no flap*	Consider prophylactic treatment in fellow eye of retinal detachment
Retinal tear	By definition caused by traction; therefore has flap or operculum	Generally requires prompt treatment unless no flashing lights and operculated, or pigmented in a patient without risk factors (phakic, no family history, etc.)
Retinoschisis	Splitting of sensory retina appears as an elevated dome most commonly inferotemporal with "snow flaking" of inner wall; usually asymptomatic; gives absolute field defect	No treatment unless break in both inner and outer layers or extension toward macula
Cobblestone	Large circular yellow lesions; may have surrounding pigment clumping; due to atrophy of pigmented epithelium	No treatment; benign

White-without-pressure	Appears as pale bands in peripheral retina; most common in blacks. May be due to vitreal retina interaction	No treatment; benign

RETINITIS PIGMENTOSA

Retinitis pigmentosa is a hereditary retinal disorder characterized by varying degrees of night blindness (nyctalopia), peripheral visual field restriction, and retinal bone corpuscular pigment clumping, especially in the peripheral retina. Other common signs include attenuation of retinal vessels, optic disc pallor, and abnormal electroretinogram (dark adapted).

Forms

- Autosomal dominant (most benign hereditary pattern)
- Autosomal recessive (most severe form)
- X-linked
- Sectorial (degeneration affects only one sector of the retina, most commonly inferior nasal, producing a corresponding visual field defect). Limited form of disease with little visual disability.
- Retinitis pigmentosa sine pigmento. Symptoms of retinitis pigmentosa without the corresponding ophthalmoscopic signs. Electroretinogram is abnormal. Pigmentary changes may appear at a later date.
- Unilateral. There is some debate as to whether this is a true retinitis pigmentosa.

Associated Disorders and Syndromes

- Laurence-Moon (Bardet-Biedl) syndrome: retinal pigmentosa, polydactyly, and adiposogenital syndrome

- Usher syndrome: retinitis pigmentosa and deafness
- Bassen-Kornzweig syndrome (hereditary abetalipoproteinemia): retinitis pigmentosa, fat intolerance, crenated erythrocytes, ataxia, and other neurologic symptoms. Perform a blood lipid profile and a peripheral blood smear to look for acanthocytes.
- Kearns-Sayre syndrome: ophthalmoplegic retinal degeneration syndrome
- Refsum's disease: retinal pigmentosa, ataxia, deafness, and progressive weakness (associated with increased serum phytanic acid)

Management

- No known effective treatment
- Rule out other conditions that may mimic retinitis pigmentosa (e.g., vitamin A deficiency, syphilis).
- Manage associated conditions (e.g., low phytol diet in Refsum's disease, management of dietary fat in Bassen-Kornzweig syndrome).
- Patient education, genetic counseling, vocational and daily living training, as necessary
- Low vision aids, night scope, etc., as needed

CENTRAL RETINAL VEIN OCCLUSION

The clinical picture of central retinal vein occlusion (CRVO) may run the gamut from just a few retinal hemorrhages and tortuous thickened retinal veins to the classic "bucket of blood" appearance with profound visual loss. The unilaterality of this condition almost always makes the differentiation from other retinopathies (e.g., diabetic) quite easy.

Clinical

Management should be directed toward preventing associated complications and detecting underlying health problems.

Medical Workup

A thorough review of past medical and ocular histories, present illness, and current use of medications is imperative. Oral contraceptives are known to be a risk factor. High blood pressure and ocular hypertension are both known to be significant contributors.

Conditions associated with CRVO include:

- Hypertension
- Diabetes mellitus
- Hyperlipidemia
- Hypercoagulability
- Hyperviscosity
- Cryofibrinogenemia
- Systemic vasculitis
- Renal disease
- Sarcoidosis
- Tuberculosis
- Leukemia
- Malignancy
- Blood dyscrasias
- Reye's syndrome
- Head injury
- Hyperuricemia
- Migraine
- Mitral valve prolapse
- Collagen vascular disease
- AIDS
- Carotid artery disease
- Elevated erythrocyte sedimentation rate
- Pregnancy
- Preeclampsia
- Platelet abnormalities
- Oral contraceptives
- Diuretics
- Sympathomimetics

A laboratory workup may include:

- Complete blood cell count and clotting factors
- SMA-18 (serum chemistries)
- Sedimentation rate
- Glucose tolerance test
- Lipid profile
- Serum protein electrophoresis
- Hemoglobin electrophoresis
- Cryoglobulins
- Serology
- Chest x-ray
- Testing for human immune deficiency virus

In addition, any history of past trauma or suspicion of an orbital mass or sinusitis may require radiologic studies of the head.

Complications

The most common complication is that of rubeotic glaucoma. Rubeotic glaucoma after CRVO is known as 90-day glaucoma because it frequently occurs about 3 months after its occurrence. It is useful to classify CRVO as ischemic or nonischemic. There is a high risk of rubeosis in the ischemic form of CRVO. Signs of ischemia include:

- Visual acuity worse than 20/100
- Severe retinopathy with multiple cotton-wool spots
- Central scotoma on Goldmann's perimetry
- Significant capillary nonperfusion on fluorescein angiography

Possession of two of the above suggests a significant risk for the future development of rubeosis. Follow initially every 1–2 weeks to rule out iris or angle neovascularization. After several weeks, nonischemic CRVOs may be followed every 1–2 months. Ischemic CRVOs should be seen at least every 2 weeks with gonioscopy at every visit for 4–6 months.

It should be kept in mind that nonischemic CRVO can convert to ischemic CRVO.

Treatment

Some physicians prescribe one baby aspirin daily in an effort to prevent further thrombus formation or reverse clotting. Anticoagulation with warfarin is not generally recommended. Thrombolysis (with streptokinase or tissue plasminogen activator) is likewise not recommended because it is associated with significant systemic risks.

The Collaborative Central Vein Occlusion Study (CVOS) demonstrated that grid laser photocoagulation is not useful for improving visual acuity reduced from macular edema. The CVOS also recommended that prophylactic panretinal photocoagulation not be performed. Panretinal photocoagulation should be promptly performed once iris or angle neovascularization is identified.

A new laser treatment for nonischemic CRVO has been described. Decreased risk of conversion to ischemic occlusion, a reduction in macular edema, and improvement in visual acuity can be achieved by using a laser to create an anastomosis between the retinal and choroidal circulations. The anastomosis was achieved by applying several spots of an argon laser (blue-green or green) over the edge of a tributary retinal vein. Typical laser settings were 50-μm spot size and a power setting of 1.5 to 2.5 watts.

BRANCH RETINAL VEIN OCCLUSION

Branch retinal vein occlusions are generally associated with a much better visual prognosis than central retinal vein occlusions. They are less likely to lead to rubeotic glaucoma and tend to show a better final visual acuity. They are characterized by sectorial regions of retinal hemorrhage and edema. Visual loss is most often a result of macular edema, secondary premacular gliosis, or capillary nonperfusion.

The most commonly affected branch of the central retinal vein is the superior temporal branch.

Management

An exhaustive search for the underlying systemic illness is usually fruitless. Most cases are due to compression by an arteriosclerotic retinal arteriole rather than primary thrombus formation. An exception, of course, is the case of a young patient with a branch retinal vein occlusion. These patients should be offered the same type of workup suggested for a CRVO. A case of previously undiagnosed systemic hypertension can be detected by measuring the blood pressure in the doctor's office.

Most cases should be given a chance to resolve on their own. A patient with a fresh occlusion should be seen every 6–8 weeks (if there are particularly large areas of capillary nonperfusion on fluorescein angiography, see the patient more frequently). Emphasis should be placed on the detection of fine neovascular vessels on the iris surface, in the angle, or on the retina. The degree of macular edema should be assessed at each visit. Retinal photocoagulation should be considered in any case in which reduced acuity from macular edema persists for longer than 6 months or if retinal or anterior segment neovascularization develops.

Branch Vein Occlusion Study

- Fifty percent of patients with macular edema from a branch retinal vein occlusion obtain visual acuity of 20/40 or better without treatment.
- Forty percent of patients with 5 DD or greater of ischemia will develop neovascularization. Neovascularization of the disc or neovascularization elsewhere usually develops within 6–12 months but can occur up to 3 years later.
- Grid laser treatment of nonclearing macular edema (3–6 months without resolution) results in a gain of two or more lines of visual acuity in 65% of patients vs. 37% of control patients.

- Sixty percent of treated eyes will have visual acuity of 20/40 or better vs. 34% of nontreated eyes.
- Twelve percent of treated eyes had visual acuities of 20/200 or worse at 3 years vs. 23% of nontreated eyes.

CENTRAL RETINAL ARTERY OCCLUSION

A central retinal artery occlusion is a true ocular emergency because permanent visual loss begins to occur just minutes after the occlusion. Patients with a fresh central retinal artery occlusion complain of severe visual loss (generally hand motions or worse, the exception being the patient with a cilioretinal artery). The retinal arterioles appear attenuated and the inner retinal layers may appear pale in contrast to the cherry-red appearance of the macula. Weeks later the arterioles may become more normal in appearance but the optic nerve will begin to atrophy.

Management

An attempt should be made to move the presumed embolus downstream, where it would cause less visual damage if the occlusion appears to have occurred within a few hours. This is accomplished through a reduction in intraocular pressure and dilation of the retinal vasculature. Each of the following has been described as a means to accomplish this:

- Digital massage: application of pressure to the globe through the eyelid for 1 minute followed by 1 minute of no pressure. Repeat several times.
- Inhalation of 5% CO_2 with 95% O_2 for 15 minutes, followed by room air for 15 minutes. Repeat for several hours.
- Paracentesis (removal of aqueous from the anterior chamber with a needle and syringe)
- Acetazolamide (injections and tablets)

An effort should be made to find the source of the embolus. If the patient appears stable, a cardiovascular consultation should be obtained. Common sources of emboli include internal carotid artery obstruction and cardiac lesions.

Other causes of central artery occlusion include giant cell arteritis, polyarteritis nodosa, and vasospasm (migraine).

Although the risk of rubeotic glaucoma is fairly low, these patients should initially be followed every 6–8 weeks during the first 6 months after the occlusion to watch for new iris vessels.

MACULAR DEGENERATION

Age-related macular degeneration (AMD) is a disease of uncertain etiology that affects older individuals, although heredity, ultraviolet radiation, nutritional deficiencies, and arteriosclerotic disease all have been suggested as contributing factors. It is the leading cause of irreversible vision loss in the United States. Known risk factors for vision loss from AMD include age, family history, cigarette smoking, hyperopia, and light iris color. It should be differentiated from hereditary macular disorders (Table 14.2).

Dry Form

- Drusen (small yellow subretinal deposits that may become confluent)
- Areas of atrophic pigment epithelial changes
- Pigment changes and clumping
- Gradual decrease in vision with minimal metamorphopsia

Vision loss may be mild to severe (legal blindness), although the majority of patients with macular degeneration with very severe vision loss have progressed to the wet (exudative) form.

Wet Form

- Choroidal neovascular membrane
- RPE detachment
- Subretinal hemorrhage/exudate

Table 14.2   Hereditary Macular Disorders

	Stargardt's	*Best's Vitelliform*	*Butterfly (Pattern)*
Inheritance	AR (also AD type)	AD	AD
Onset of symptoms	First to second decades	First decade	Second to fifth decades
Clinical findings	Beaten bronze appearance in macular region often with para-foveal flecks	Vitelliform (sunnyside up) lesion early; may progress to scrambled egg/ atrophy and neovascular-ization	Reticular pattern of pigmentation; propeller-like appearance
Degree of visual dis-ability	Severe (<20/200)	Surprisingly good vision with vitel-liform lesion; may progress to 20/30 to 20/50; rarely 20/200	Mild to moderate visual acuity loss (20/25 to 20/70)

AD = autosomal dominant; AR = autosomal recessive.

- More rapid vision loss, often with metamorphopsia (distortion of straight lines)

Management of the Dry Form

- Careful examination with Amsler grid testing and detailed examination looking for exudative lesions
- Patients should be instructed in self-monitoring with Amsler grid. Changes in vision and metamorphopsia should be reported promptly.
- At present there is no accepted treatment for the dry form of macular degeneration. Oral vitamin and zinc supplements have been advocated by some physicians. Also ultraviolet ray protection is advised.

Management of the Wet Form

- Amsler grid test with detailed funduscopic examination
- Fluorescein angiography for those lesions determined to be potentially treatable (absence of subretinal scarring)
- Prompt laser photocoagulation for treatable subretinal membranes
- Surgical removal of foveal subretinal membranes is being investigated
- Low vision aids can be beneficial to those with a visual disability that cannot be treated.

OCULAR HISTOPLASMOSIS SYNDROME

The fungus *Histoplasma capsulatum* is responsible for a multifocal choroiditis most commonly seen in patients who have lived or visited the Mississippi River or Ohio River valley regions. Vision loss may occur as a result of choroidal neovascular membrane formation. Choroidal neovascularization usually, but not invariably, will occur in association with a chorioretinal scar in the posterior pole.

Signs and Symptoms

- Small, round, atrophic, "punched out" chorioretinal scars in the midperipheral retina and posterior pole
- Peripapillary chorioretinal scarring
- No vitreous or anterior chamber reaction
- Choroidal neovascularization in a minority of patients

Management

- Skin testing to confirm the diagnosis is generally not performed.
- Laser photocoagulation for treatable choroidal neovascularization
- Amsler grid monitoring for patients with posterior pole or peripapillary scarring

Table 14.3   Causes of Choroidal Neovascularization

Age-related macular degeneration
Ocular histoplasmosis
Idiopathic
High myopia
Photocoagulation scars
Choroidal rupture
Angioid streaks
Hereditary macular dystrophies
Retinitis pigmentosa
Following choroiditis
Choroidal nevus
Choroidal melanoma
Other choroidal tumors; primary or metastatic
Optic pits
Choroidal colobomas
Central serous choroidopathy
Retinal vein occlusions

CHOROIDAL NEOVASCULARIZATION

When neovascular membranes grow through Bruch's membrane into the subpigment epithelial or subretinal space, they may produce leakage of fluid and blood with subsequent pigment epithelial detachment, scarring, and profound loss of central vision. Table 14.3 lists conditions known to be associated with choroidal neovascularization (CNV). The most common cause of CNV is AMD, but any condition that affects the integrity of Bruch's membrane and/or the RPE may predispose to it.

Signs and Symptoms

- Sudden loss of visual acuity
- Central scotoma or metamorphopsia
- Subretinal fluid or hemorrhage
- Gray or green subretinal lesion

- Pigment epithelial detachment
- Often with subretinal or intraretinal lipid
- Later the lesion may take on the appearance of a disciform scar or massive subretinal lipid accumulation (senile coats).

Management

- Fluorescein angiogram to identify the net. The neovascularization may be well defined or "occult" due to poor transmission through overlying fluid or blood.
- The Macular Photocoagulation Study demonstrated the effectiveness of laser photocoagulation in preventing severe vision loss. This should be offered promptly to patients with treatable nets.
- Treatments currently under investigation include subretinal thrombolysis and surgical removal of membranes or scars.
- Fellow eyes and previously affected eyes should be monitored with Amsler grids.
- Low vision aids can be of benefit to patients affected with significant vision loss.

DIABETIC RETINOPATHY

Diabetic retinopathy is the leading cause of blindness in patients 25–74 years of age. A simple way to classify diabetic retinopathy that has important management implications is to subdivide it into a nonproliferative (background) form and a proliferative form.

Background diabetic retinopathy is characterized by intraretinal microaneurysms, hemorrhages, nerve fiber layer infarcts (cotton-wool spots), hard exudates, and microvascular anomalies. It can be described in terms of grades that have been established to document severity and risk. Table 14.4 presents a management scheme based on the severity of retinopathy.

The most severe grade of background diabetic retinopathy is pre-proliferative diabetic retinopathy.

Proliferative diabetic retinopathy obtains its name from the proliferation of new blood vessels (neovascularization). It is sometimes associated with accompanying fibrous tissue.

Table 14.4 Diabetic Retinopathy

Stage of Retinopathy	Clinical Signs	Management
Background retinopathy	Microaneurysms, hemorrhages, hard exudates	Follow every 6–12 mos
Preproliferative retinopathy	Beaded veins, cotton-wool spots, intra-retinal microvas-cular anomalies	Follow every 2–4 mos
Proliferative retinopathy	Neovascularization of the disc, neovas-cularization else-where, preretinal or vitreous hemorrhage	Panretinal photocoagulation
Rubeosis iridis	Neovascularization of iris	Panretinal photocoagulation; cyclocryotherapy or other measures may be required for uncontrolled glaucoma

Note: Macular edema or hard exudates threatening the fovea may require focal or grid photocoagulation.

By ophthalmoscopy, proliferative retinopathy manifests itself as fine, branching blood vessels that grow into the vitreous. These vessels are best seen by the use of a fundus contact lens or indirect condensing lens.

Neovascularization shows profuse leakage on fluorescein angiography. Vitreous hemorrhage from neovascularization may obscure the underlying proliferative vessels.

Examination of the iris for rubeosis (neovascularization) should be performed on all diabetic patients.

The Diabetes Control and Complications Trial confirmed that intensive treatment for blood glucose control has profound benefits in terms of reducing the development and risk of progression of diabetic retinopathy.

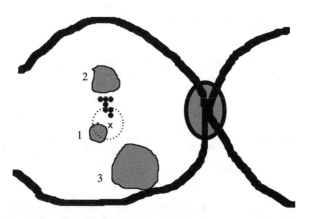

Fig. 14.1   Clinically significant macular edema. 1. Retinal thickening within 500 μm of the center of the fovea. 2. Hard exudates within 500 μm of the center of the fovea associated with retinal thickening. 3. Retinal edema > 1 disc area in size and within 1 DD of the center of the fovea.

The Early Treatment Diabetic Retinopathy Study (ETDRS) confirmed that clinically significant macular edema benefited from focal argon laser coagulation.

Clinically Significant Macular Edema (CSME)

- Thickening of the retina at or within 500 μm of the center of the macula as judged by slit-lamp biomicroscopy
- Hard exudate at or within 500 μm of the center of the macula associated with thickening of the adjacent retina
- Retinal thickening 1 DD or larger, part of which is within 1 DD of the center of the macula (Fig. 14.1)

Nonproliferative Retinopathy Management

- The principal mechanism of vision loss in nonproliferative retinopathy is through macular edema.
- Macular edema may develop from focal vascular leakage, which may be treated with focal laser photocoagulation.
- More diffuse vascular leakage may also result in macular edema. Diffuse leakage is typically treated with grid photocoagulation.
- Detection of macular edema requires stereoscopic examination of the retina by slit-lamp biomicroscopy and manifests as retinal thickening.
- Fluorescein angiography is generally performed before laser photocoagulation to delineate sources of leakage.
- More severe diabetic retinopathy may require more frequent follow-up.
- Retinal photography may be helpful in detecting and documenting retinopathy.

Proliferative Retinopathy Management

- Proliferative retinopathy may produce vision loss through traction retinal detachment or vitreous hemorrhage.
- Panretinal laser photocoagulation is indicated for proliferative retinopathy. It may cause regression of neovascularization.
- Patients with high-risk characteristics are especially at risk for severe vision loss and should receive panretinal photocoagulation promptly (Fig. 14.2).
- If possible, focal photocoagulation to treat CSME should be performed before panretinal photocoagulation. Panretinal photocoagulation can lead to or exacerbate macular edema.
- Krypton red is scattered less by media opacities and may be preferable when vitreous hemorrhage or cataract is present.
- Vitrectomy is indicated for nonclearing vitreous hemorrhage, bilateral vitreous hemorrhage impairing vision, loculated premacular hemorrhage, combined traction and rhegmatogenous retinal detachment, or macular detachment or distortion from traction.

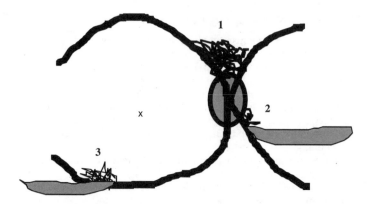

Fig. 14.2   High-risk characteristics. 1. Neovascularization of the disc ¼–⅓ disc area in size or larger. 2. Any neovascularization of the disc with preretinal or vitreous hemorrhage. 3. Neovascularization elsewhere greater than ½ disc area in size associated with preretinal or vitreous hemorrhage.

High-Risk Proliferative Retinopathy Characteristics

- Mild neovascularization of the disc with vitreous hemorrhage
- Moderate to severe neovascularization of the disc without hemorrhage
- Moderate to severe neovascularization of the disc with vitreous hemorrhage
- Moderate to severe neovascularization of the disc elsewhere with vitreous hemorrhage

SICKLE CELL RETINOPATHY

Intravascular sickling of red blood cells can lead to vascular occlusions, capillary nonperfusion, retinal ischemia, and retinal neovascularization.

Sickle cell disease afflicts 0.4% of African Americans. Sickle trait is found in 8% of African Americans.

Retinal neovascularization, vitreous hemorrhage, and retinal detachment are more commonly found in SC disease than sickle cell disease or sickle cell trait.

The peripheral retina is the sight of most of the ocular pathology associated with the sickling disorders.

Signs and Symptoms

- Salmon patch hemorrhages, which are intraretinal hemorrhages associated with peripheral retinal arteriolar occlusions
- Black sunburst lesions, which are areas of RPE hyperplasia/hypertrophy and are usually perivascular in location
- Refractile spots that are resorbed hemorrhages within acquired schisis cavities
- Sea fans (neovascularization), which may autoinfarct
- Vitreous hemorrhage
- Traction and rhegmatogenous retinal detachments

Treatment

- Segmental scatter photocoagulation for sea fans
- Surgery for retinal detachment or nonclearing vitreal hemorrhage
- There is a risk of anterior segment ischemia and necrosis in association with scleral buckling surgery.

VON HIPPEL-LINDAU DISEASE AND ANGIOMATOSIS RETINAE

Angiomatosis retinae is a condition characterized by the formation of retinal capillary hemangiomas. Capillary hemangiomas appear as spherical orange or red tumors fed by a dilated, tortuous retinal artery and drained by an engorged vein. The lesions are bilateral in 50% of patients. Small lesions are easily overlooked. Leakage from the angiomas may result in macular edema, hard exudates in the macula, serous retinal detachments, or vitreous hemorrhage. When capillary hemangiomas are associated with central nervous system or visceral disease, the condition is termed von Hippel-Lindau disease. Angiomatosis retinae exists in both a hereditary (autosomal dominant) form and a sporadic form.

Associated Lesions in Von Hippel-Lindau Disease

- Retinal capillary hemangiomas
- Posterior fossa/cerebellar hemangioblastomas
- Spinal hemangioblastomas
- Pancreatic and renal tumors or cysts
- Liver, epididymal, or ovarian cysts
- Renal cell carcinoma
- Polycythemia
- Adrenal medullary pheochromocytomas

Management

- Photocoagulation, cryotherapy, or diathermy of capillary hemangiomas. Photocoagulation of the feeding retinal artery can be used to successfully manage these lesions.
- A search for central nervous system and systemic lesions should be initiated.
- Careful follow-up is necessary to detect new retinal lesions.

CYTOMEGALOVIRUS RETINITIS

Cytomegalovirus (CMV) is the most common opportunistic ocular infection in AIDS patients. Patients with CD4+ T cell counts less than 100 cells/µl are especially at risk for the infection.

Signs and Symptoms

- Yellowish white areas of retinal opacification with irregular borders often with associated hemorrhage (appearance of "crumbled cheese and ketchup").

- Low-grade iritis or vitritis
- Small, early CMV lesions may occasionally be confused with a cotton-wool spot. See the patient back in 1 week. The rapid progression of CMV retinopathy generally resolves the confusion.
- Patients may complain of decreased vision or new floaters but may be asymptomatic.
- There is a high incidence of rhegmatogenous retinal detachment.

Management

- Patients with CD4+ counts under 100 cells/µl should be screened for CMV retinitis every 3–6 months and be advised to report visual symptoms immediately.
- Patients with active retinitis should be seen at least monthly.
- Fundus photography and retinal drawings should be used to monitor patients.
- Medical treatment generally consists of the following:
  1. Foscarnet sodium, 90 mg/kg IV q12h induction for 2 weeks, followed by a maintenance dose of 120 mg/kg IV daily. Main side effects are nephrotoxicity and hypercalcemia.
  2. Ganciclovir sodium, 5 mg/kg q12h induction for 2 weeks, followed by a maintenance dose of 10 mg/kg IV or 1,000 mg PO three times a day. The main side effect is hematologic suppression.
  3. Cidofovir dihydrate 5 mg/kg IV once a week for 2 weeks induction, followed by 3–5 mg/kg IV maintenance every 2 weeks. Hydration with 1–2 liters of saline before cidofovir administration and probenecid, 4 g over 8 hours, may limit nephrotoxicity. Nephrotoxicity, neutropenia, peripheral neuropathy, iritis, and ocular hypotony are potential side effects.
- Virus resistance may require combination drug therapy.
- Systemic side effects may warrant intravitreal injections. Induction is with ganciclovir, 200 µg/0.1 ml, or foscarnet, 1,200 µg/0.1 ml, twice a week. Reduce to once a week for maintenance.
- IV injections of cidofovir, 20 µg/0.1 ml every 5–6 weeks, have also been described. Oral probenecid, 2 g 3 hours before and 1 g given 2

and 8 hours after injection, was used in an effort to decrease the possibility of a toxic effect. Ocular hypotony occurred in 3% of patients.

- Fomivirsen is a new drug undergoing clinical trials for CMV retinitis.
- Rhegmatogenous retinal detachments generally require vitrectomy with silicone oil.

NOTES

15

Conversion Charts and Laboratory Testing

Table 15.1 Vertex Distance Conversion Chart*

Spectacle power	Plus Lenses' Vertex Distance		Minus Lenses' Vertex Distance	
	10 mm	14 mm	10 mm	14 mm
4.00	4.12	4.25	3.87	3.75
4.50	4.75	4.75	4.25	4.25
5.00	5.25	5.37	4.75	4.62
5.50	5.75	6.00	5.25	5.12
6.00	6.37	6.50	5.62	5.50
6.50	7.00	7.12	6.12	6.00
7.00	7.50	7.75	6.50	6.37
7.50	8.12	8.37	7.00	6.75
8.00	8.75	9.00	7.37	7.25
8.50	9.25	9.62	7.87	7.62
9.00	9.87	10.37	8.25	8.00
9.50	10.50	11.00	8.62	8.37
10.00	11.12	11.62	9.12	8.75
10.50	11.75	12.25	9.50	9.12
11.00	12.37	13.00	9.87	9.50
11.50	13.00	13.75	10.37	9.87
12.00	13.62	14.50	10.75	10.25
12.50	14.25	15.25	11.12	10.62
13.00	15.00	16.00	11.50	11.00
13.50	15.62	16.62	11.87	11.37
14.00	16.25	17.50	12.25	11.75

(continued on p. 210)

Table 15.1   (continued)

Spectacle power	Plus Lenses' Vertex Distance		Minus Lenses' Vertex Distance	
	10 mm	14 mm	10 mm	14 mm
14.50	17.00	18.25	12.62	12.00
15.00	17.75	19.00	13.00	12.37
15.50	18.25	19.75	13.50	12.75
16.00	19.00	20.50	13.75	13.00
16.50	19.75	21.50	14.12	13.50
17.00	20.50	22.25	14.50	13.75
17.50	21.25	23.25	14.87	14.00
18.00	22.00	24.00	15.25	14.37
18.50	22.75	25.00	15.62	14.75
19.00	23.50	26.00	16.00	15.00

*The chart describes changes in power needed to go from spectacle correction to contact lens correction (and vice versa). For example, a patient wearing a –7.00 in a spectacle lens positioned 10 mm in front of the eye would require a –6.50 contact lens correction.

Table 15.2 Keratometer Conversion Chart

Diopter (mm)	Diopter (mm)	Diopter (mm)
36.00 (9.38)	44.00 (7.67)	52.00 (6.49)
36.25 (9.31)	44.25 (7.63)	52.25 (6.46)
36.50 (9.25)	44.50 (7.58)	52.50 (6.43)
36.75 (9.18)	44.75 (7.54)	52.75 (6.40)
37.00 (9.12)	45.00 (7.50)	53.00 (6.37)
37.25 (9.06)	45.25 (7.46)	53.25 (6.34)
37.50 (9.00)	45.50 (7.42)	53.50 (6.31)
37.75 (8.94)	45.75 (7.38)	53.75 (6.28)
38.00 (8.88)	46.00 (7.34)	54.00 (6.25)
38.25 (8.82)	46.25 (7.30)	54.25 (6.50)
38.50 (8.77)	46.50 (7.26)	54.50 (6.19)
38.75 (8.71)	46.75 (7.22)	54.75 (6.16)
39.00 (8.65)	47.00 (7.18)	55.00 (6.14)
39.25 (8.60)	47.25 (7.14)	55.25 (6.11)
39.50 (8.54)	47.50 (7.11)	55.50 (6.08)
39.75 (8.49)	47.75 (7.07)	55.75 (6.05)
40.00 (8.44)	48.00 (7.03)	56.00 (6.03)
40.25 (8.39)	48.25 (6.99)	56.25 (6.00)
40.50 (8.33)	48.50 (6.96)	36.50 (5.97)
40.75 (8.28)	48.75 (6.92)	56.75 (5.95)
41.00 (8.23)	49.00 (6.89)	57.00 (5.92)
41.25 (8.18)	49.25 (6.85)	57.25 (5.90)
41.50 (8.13)	49.50 (6.82)	57.50 (5.87)
41.75 (8.08)	49.75 (6.78)	57.75 (5.84)
42.00 (8.04)	50.00 (6.75)	58.00 (5.82)
42.25 (7.99)	50.25 (6.72)	58.25 (5.79)
42.50 (7.94)	50.50 (6.68)	58.50 (5.77)
42.75 (7.89)	50.75 (6.65)	58.75 (5.75)
43.00 (7.85)	51.00 (6.62)	59.00 (5.72)
43.25 (7.80)	51.25 (6.59)	59.25 (5.70)
43.50 (7.76)	51.50 (6.55)	59.50 (5.67)
43.75 (7.71)	51.75 (6.52)	59.75 (5.65)

Table 15.3   Keratometer Extended Range

+1.25		−1.00	
Drum reading	Corneal power	Drum reading	Corneal power
43.00	50.134	36.00	30.874
43.25	50.425	36.25	31.088
43.50	50.176	36.50	31.302
43.75	51.007	36.75	31.516
44.00	51.298	37.00	31.730
44.25	51.589	37.25	31.944
44.50	51.880	37.50	32.158
44.75	52.171	37.75	32.372
45.00	52.462	38.00	32.586
45.25	52.753	38.25	32.800
45.50	53.044	38.50	33.014
45.75	53.335	38.75	33.228
46.00	53.626	39.00	33.447
46.25	53.917	39.25	33.661
46.50	54.208	39.50	33.875
46.75	54.499	39.75	34.089
47.00	54.790	40.00	34.303
47.25	55.081	40.25	34.517
47.50	55.380	40.50	34.731
47.75	55.671	40.75	34.945
48.00	55.962	41.00	35.159
48.25	56.253	41.25	35.373
48.50	56.544	41.50	35.587
48.75	56.835	41.75	35.801
49.00	57.126		
49.25	57.417		
49.50	57.708		
49.75	57.999		
50.00	58.290		
50.25	58.581		
50.50	58.872		
50.75	59.163		
51.00	59.454		
51.25	59.745		
51.50	60.036		
51.75	60.327		

Table 15.4   Metric Weight Conversions

kg	lb	kg	lb	kg	lb
1	2.2	45	99	90	198
5	11	50	110	95	209
10	22	55	121	100	220
15	33	60	132	105	231
20	44	65	143	110	242
25	55	70	154	115	253
30	66	75	165	120	264
35	77	80	176	125	275
40	88	85	187	130	286

Table 15.5   Metric Conversions

When You Know	Multiply By	To Find
Millimeters (mm)	0.04	Inches (in)
Centimeters (cm)	0.4	Inches (in)
Meters (m)	3.3	Feet (ft)
Meters (m)	1.1	Yards (yd)
Kilometers (km)	0.62	Miles (mi)
Grams (gm)	0.035	Ounces (oz)
Kilograms (kg)	2.2	Pounds (lb)
Milliliters (ml)	0.2	Teaspoons (tsp)

Table 15.6   Laboratory Testing: Typical Normal Reference Ranges

Test	Normal Ranges
Hematologic	
Bleeding time	2–7 min
Hematocrit	
Male	42–52%
Female	38–47%
Hemoglobin	
Male	13.5–18.0 g/dl
Female	12.0–16.0 g/dl
MCV	80–96 m^2/RBC
MCH(C)	32–36 g/dl
MCH	27–32 pg
Erythrocyte count	
Male	$4.3–6.2 \times 10^6$/µl
Female	$3.5–5.4 \times 10^6$/µl
WBC	$4.5–11.0 \times 10^3$/µl
White cell differential	
Segmented neutrophils	1800–7000/µl (51–67%)
Bands	0–700/µl (<10%)
Eosinophils	0–450/µl (2–4%)
Basophils	0–200/µl (0–1%)
Lymphocytes	1000–4800/µl (21–35%)
Monocytes	0–800/µl (4–8%)
Platelet count	150,000–450,000/mm^3
PT	11.0–13.5 sec
PTT	27–38 sec
Reticulocyte count	0.5–1.5% of RBC
Sedimentation rate	
(Westergren)	
Male	0–15 mm/hr
Female	0–20 mm/hr

Test	Normal Ranges
Blood chemistry	
Albumin	3.5–5.0 g/dl
Alkaline phosphatase	20–90 U/liter
ALT, GPT	8–20 U/liter
AST, GOT	8–20 U/liter
Bilirubin (adult): total/direct	0.1–1.0/0.0–0.3 mg/dl
Calcium	8.4–10.2 mg/dl
Cholesterol	120–200 mg/dl
Creatinine	0.5–1.4 mg/dl
Electrolytes	
Sodium	135–147 mEq/liter
Chloride	95–105 mEq/liter
Potassium	3.5–5.0 mEq/liter
Bicarbonate	22–28 mEq/liter
Fibrinogen	177–375 mg/dl
Glucose	
Fasting	70–110 mg/dl
2-hr postprandial	<120 mg/dl
LDH	200–450 U/ml
Phosphorus	3.0–4.5 mg/dl
Total protein	6.0–7.8 g/dl
Triglycerides	30–160 mg/dl
T_3	115–190 ng/dl
T_4	5–12 µg/dl
TSH	0.5–10 µU/ml
Urea nitrogen	7–18 mg/dl
Uric acid	3.0–8.2 mg/dl

MCV = mean corpuscular volume; MCH(C) = mean corpuscular hemoglobin (concentration); WBC = white blood cell (count); RBC = red blood cell (count); PT = prothrombin time; PTT = partial thromboplastin time; ALT = alanine transaminase; GPT = glutamic pyruvic transaminase; AST = aspartate transaminase; GOT = glutamic-oxaloacetic transaminase; LDH = lactic dehydrogenase; T_3 = triiodothyronine; T_4 = thyroxine; TSH = thyroid-stimulating hormone.

16

Trade Names and Generic Names of Commonly Prescribed Medications

Trade Name	Generic Name
Accupril	Quinapril hydrochloride
Accutane	Isotretinoin
Achromycin V	Tetracycline
Actifed	Pseudoephedrine hydrochloride, triprolidine
Actifed-C	Codeine phosphate, guaifenesin, pseudoephedrine hydrochloride, triprolidine hydrochloride
Adapin	Doxepin hydrochloride
Aldactazide	Spironolactone, hydrochlorothiazide
Aldactone	Spironolactone
Aldomet	Methyldopa
Aldoril	Methyldopa, hydrochlorothiazide
Altace	Ramipril
Alupent	Metaproterenol
Ambien	Zolpidem tartrate
Amcill	Ampicillin
Amoxicillin	Amoxicillin
Amoxil	Amoxicillin
Anaprox	Naproxen sodium
Ancef	Cefazolin

Trade Name	*Generic Name*
Ansaid	Flurbiprofen
Antabuse	Disulfiram
Antivert	Meclizine
Anturane	Sulfinpyrazone
Apresazide	Hydrazaline, hydrochlorothiazide
Apresoline	Hydralazine
Atarax	Hydroxyzine hydrochloride
Ativan	Lorazepam
Atromid-S	Clofibrate
Augmentin	Amoxicillin/clavulanate
AVC Cream	Sulfanilamide
Aventyl	Nortriptyline
Axid	Nizatidine
Azulfidine	Sulfasalazine
Bactrim	Trimethoprim-sulfamethaxazole
Benadryl	Diphenhydramine
Bendectin	Doxylamine succinate, pyridoxine hydrochloride
Benemid	Probenicid
Bentyl	Dicyclomine
Benylin	Ammonium chloride, diphenhydramine hydrochloride, sodium citrate
Betapace	Sotalol hydrochloride
Biaxin	Clarithromycin
Blocadren	Timolol maleate
Brethine	Terbutaline sulfate
Brevibloc	Esmolol hydrochloride
Bumex	Bumetanide
BuSpar	Buspirone hydrochloride
Butazolidin alka	Phenylbutazone
Butisol sodium	Butabarbitol
Calan	Verapamil hydrochloride
Capoten	Captopril

Trade Name	Generic Name
Carafate	Sucralfate
Cardene	Nicardipine hydrochloride
Cardizem	Diltiazem hydrochloride
Cardura	Doxazosin mesylate
Catapres	Clonidine
Ceclor	Cefaclor
Cefobid	Cefaperazone
Ceftin	Cefuroxime axetil
Cefzil	Cefprozil
Centrax	Prazepam
Chloromycetin	Chloramphenicol
Chlor-Trimeton	Chlorpheniramine maleate
Choledyl	Oxtriphylline
Chronulac	Lactulose
Cipro	Ciprofloxacin
Claforan	Cefotaxime
Claritin	Loratadine
Cleocin	Clindamycin
Clinoril	Sulindac
Clonopin	Clonazepam
Clozaril	Clozapine
Cogentin	Benztropine mesylate
Colestid	Colestipol
Combid	Isopromadine, prochlorperazine
Compazine	Phenothiazine
Corgard	Nadolol
Cordarone	Amiodarone
Coumadin	Warfarin sodium
Dalmane	Flurazepam
Danocrine	Danazol
Dantrium	Dantrolene sodium
Dapsone USP	Dapsone
Darvocet-N	Propoxyphene napsylate, acetaminophen

Trade Name	Generic Name
Darvon	Propoxyphene hydrochloride
Darvon Compound-65	Propoxyphene hydrochloride, caffeine, aspirin
Daypro	Oxaprozin
Decadron	Dexamethasone
Declomycin	Demeclocycline hydrochloride
Deltasone	Prednisone
Demulen	Oral contraceptive
Depakene/Depakote	Valproic acid, divalproex
Desyrel	Trazadone
Diabeta	Glyburide
Diabinese	Chlorpropamide
Didronel	Etidronate disodium
DiFlucon	Fluconazole
Dilantin	Phenytoin
Dilaudid	Hydromorphone hydrochloride
Dimetapp	Brompheniramine, phenylephrine, phenyl-propanolamine
Ditropan	Oxybutynin chloride
Diuril	Chlorothiazide
Dobutrex	Dobutamine
Dolobid	Diflunisal
Dolophine	Methadone
Donnatal	Atropine sulfate, hyoscine hydrobromide, hyoscyamine, phenobarbital
Dramamine	Dimenhydrinate
Drixoral	Dexbrompheniramine maleate, pseudoephedrine sulfate
Duricef	Cefadroxil monohydrate
Dyazide	Hydrochlorothiazide, triamterene
Dymelor	Acetohexamide
Dynapen	Dicloxacillin sodium
E.E.S.	Erythromycin

Trade Name	Generic Name
E-Mycin	Erythromycin
Elavil	Amitriptyline
Eldepryl	Selegiline hydrochloride
Empirin with codeine	Aspirin with codeine
Enduron	Methyclothiazide
Equagesic	Meprobamate, aspirin
Ergostat	Ergotamine tartrate
Ergotrate Maleate	Ergonovine maleate
Erythromycin	Erythromycin
Esidrix	Hydrochlorothiazide
Estrace	Estradiol
Feldene	Piroxicam
Fiorinal	Butalbital, aspirin, caffeine
Fiorinal with codeine	Codeine, codeine phosphate, butalbital, caffeine, aspirin
Flagyl	Metronidazole
Flexeril	Cyclobenzaprine
Floxin	Ofloxacin
Gantrisin	Sulfisoxazole
Glucotrol	Glipizide
Glynase PresTab	Glyburide micronized
Grisactin	Griseofulvin
Gyne-Lotrimin	Clotrimazole
Halcion	Triazolam
Haldol	Haloperidol
Hismanal	Astemizole
Hydergine	Ergot alkaloids
Hydrochlorothiazide	Hydrochlorothiazide
Hydrodiuril	Hydrochlorothiazide
Hydropres	Reserpine, hydrochlorothiazide
Hygroton	Chlorthalidone
Hytrin	Terazosin hydrochloride
Ilosone	Erythromycin

Trade Name	Generic Name
Imodium	Loperamide
Imuran	Azathioprine
Inderal	Propanolol hydrochloride
Indocin	Indomethacin
Inocor	Amrinone
Ionamin	Phentermine hydrochloride
Ismo	Isosorbide mononitrate
Isoptin	Verapamil hydrochloride
Isopto Carpine	Pilocarpine ophthalmic solution
Isordil	Isosorbide dinitrate
K-Lor	Potassium chloride
K-Lyte	Potassium chloride
K-Tab	Potassium chloride
Keflex	Cephalexin
Keflin	Cephalothin
Kefzol	Cefazolin
Kenalog	Triamcinolone acetonide
Klonopin	Clonazepam
Kwell	Gamma benzene hexachloride
Lanoxin	Digoxin
Larotid	Amoxicillin
Lasix	Furosemide
Ledercillin VK	Penicillin V
Librax	Chlordiazepoxide hydrochloride, clidinium bromide
Librium	Chlordiazepoxide
Lidex	Fluocininide
Limbitrol	Chlordiazepoxide, amitriptyline hydrochloride
Lodine	Etodolac
Lomotil	Atropine sulfate, diphenoxylate
Loniten	Minoxidil
Lo/Ovral	Oral contraceptive

Trade Name	Generic Name
Lopid	Gemfibrozil
Lopressor	Metoprolol
Lorabid	Loracarbef
Lorelco	Probucol
Lotensin	Benazepril hydrochloride
Lotrimin	Clotrimazole
Lozol	Indapamide
Ludiomol	Maprotilene
Macrobid	Nitrofurantoin
Macrodantin	Nitrofurantoin
Marezine	Cyclizine
Maxzide	Triamterene, hydrochlorothiazide
Mellaril	Thioridazine hydrochloride
Meclomen	Meclofenamate sodium
Medrol	Methylprednisolone
Mestinon	Pyridostigmine bromide
Mevacor	Lovastatin
Mexitil	Mexiletine hydrochloride
Micronase	Glyburide
Midamor	Amiloride
Minipress	Prazosin
Minocin	Minocycline
Modicon	Oral contraceptive
Monistat	Miconazole nitrate
Motrin	Ibuprofen
Mycolog	Nystatin, triamcinolone
Mysoline	Primidone
Naldecon	Phenylpropanolamine hydrochloride, phenylephrine hydrochloride, phenyltoloxamine citrate, chlorpheniramine maleate
Nalfon	Fenoprofen calcium
Naprosyn	Naproxen

Trade Name	Generic Name
Navane	Thiothixene
Nebcin	Tobramycin
Nicolar	Niacin
Nipride	Nitroprusside
Nitro-Bid	Nitroglycerin
Nitroglycerin	Nitroglycerin
Nitrol	Nitroglycerin
Nitrostat	Nitroglycerin
Nizoral	Ketoconazole
Nolvadex	Tamoxifen
Norgesic Forte	Orphenadrine citrate, aspirin, caffeine
Norinyl	Oral contraceptive
Normodyne	Labetalol
Norpace	Disopyramide phosphate
Norpramin	Desipramine
Norvasc	Amlodipine besylate
Omnipen	Ampicillin
Orinase	Tolbutamide
Ornade	Phenylpropanolamine, chlorpheniramine maleate
Ortho-Novum	Oral contraceptive
Orudis	Ketoprofen
Ovral	Oral contraceptive
Ovulen	Oral contraceptive
Pamelor	Nortriptyline hydrochloride
Parafon Forte	Chlorzoxazone
Pathocil	Dicloxacillin sodium
Pavabid	Papaverine
Penicillin VK	Penicillin V
Pen-Vee K	Penicillin V
Pepcid	Famotidine
Percocet-5	Oxycodone hydrochloride, acetaminophen
Percodan	Oxycodone hydrochloride, oxycodone terephthalate, aspirin

Trade Name	Generic Name
Periactin	Cyproheptadine hydrochloride
Persantine	Dipyridamole
Pfizerpen A	Ampicillin
Pfizerpen VK	Penicillin V
Phenaphen with codeine	Acetaminophen
Phenergan Syrup	Promethazine hydrochloride, alcohol
Phenergan with codeine	Codeine phosphate, promethazine hydrochloride
Phenergan VC with codeine	Codeine phosphate, promethazine hydrochloride, phenylephrine hydrochloride, alcohol
Phenobarbital	Phenobarbital
Poly-Vi-Flor	Multivitamin, sodium fluoride
Pravachol	Pravastatin sodium
Premarin	Conjugated estrogens
Prilosec	Omeprazole
Principen	Ampicillin
Prinivil	Lisinopril
Procan SR	Procainamide
Procardia	Nifedipine
Prolixin	Fluphenazine hydrochloride
Pronestyl	Procainamide
Proscar	Finasteride
Prostigmin	Neostigmine bromide
Proventil	Albuterol
Provera	Medroxyprogesterone
Prozac	Fluoxetine hydrochloride
Pyridium	Phenazopyridine hydrochloride
Questran	Cholestyramine
Quinex	Quinidine
Reglan	Metoclopramide
Relafen	Nabumetone

Trade Name	Generic Name
Restoril	Temazepam
Retrovir	AZT
Rifadin	Rifampin
Ritalin	Methylphenidate
Robaxin	Methocarbamol
Rythmol	Propafenone hydrochloride
Sandimmine	Cyclosporine
Sansert	Methysergide maleate
Seldane	Terfenadine
Septra	Trimethoprim-sulfamethoxazole
Septra DS	Trimethoprim-sulfamethoxazole
Ser-Ap-ES	Reserpine, hydralazine hydrochloride, hydrochlorothiazide
Serax	Oxazepam
Sinemet	Carbidopa, levodopa
Sinequan	Doxepin hydrochloride
SK-Ampicillin	Ampicillin
Slo-Bid	Theophylline anhydrous
Slo-Phyllin	Theophylline
Slow-K	Potassium chloride
Sodium Sulamyd	Sulfacetamide sodium
Soma	Carisoprodol
Sorbitrate	Isosorbide dinitrate
Spectrobid	Bacampicillin hydrochloride
Stadol	Butorphanol tartrate
Stelazine	Trifluoperazine
Stuartnatal 1 + 1	Multivitamin, multimineral
Sudafed	Pseudoephedrine
Sumycin	Tetracycline
Suprax	Cefixime
Symmetrel	Amantadine hydrochloride
Synalgos-DC	Drocode bitartrate, aspirin, caffeine
Synthroid	Levothyroxine sodium

Trade Name	Generic Name
Tagamet	Cimetidine
Talwin	Pentazocine
Tavist	Clemastine fumarate
Tegretol	Carbamazepine
Tenormin	Atenolol
Tenuate	Diethylpropion hydrochloride
Tetracycline	Tetracycline
Theo-Dur	Theophylline
Thorazine	Chlorpromazine
Thyroid	Thyroid hormone
Ticlid	Ticlopidine hydrochloride
Tigan	Trimethobenzamide hydrochloride
Timoptic	Timolol
Tofranil	Imipramine
Tolectin	Tolmetin sodium
Tolinase	Tolazamide
Tonocard	Tocainide hydrochloride
Topicort	Desoximetasone
Tranxene	Clorazepate
Triavil	Perphenazine, amitriptyline hydrochloride
Trimox	Amoxicillin
Tussionex	Hydrocone, phenyltoloxamine
Tuss-Ornade	Caramiphen edisylate, chlorpheniramine maleate, isopropamide iodide, phenylpropanolamine hydrochloride
Tylenol with codeine	Acetaminophen with codeine
Unisom	Doxylamine succinate
Urecholine	Bethanechol chloride
V-Cillin K	Penicillin V
Valisone	Betamethasone
Valium	Diazepam
Vanceril	Beclomethasone
Vantin	Cefpodoxime

Trade Name	Generic Name
Vasotec	Enalapril
Veetids	Penicillin V
Ventolin	Albuterol
Viagra	Sildenafil citrate
Vibramycin	Doxycycline
Vibra-Tab	Doxycycline
Vistaril	Hydroxyzine hydrochloride
Vitravene	Fomivirsen
Vivactil	Protriptyline
Voltaren	Diclofenac sodium
Wellbutrin	Bupropion hydrochloride
Wymox	Amoxicillin
Wytensin	Guanabenz
Xanax	Alprazolam
Zantac	Ranitidine
Zarontin	Ethosuximide
Zaroxolyn	Metolazone
Zestril	Lisinopril
Zithromax	Azithromycin dihydrate
Zocor	Simvastatin
Zoloft	Sertraline hydrochloride
Zomax	Zomepirac
Zovirax	Acyclovir
Zyloprim	Allopurinol

NOTES

17

Ocular Side Effects of Pharmaceutical Agents

ANISOCORIA

Alcohol
Brompheniramine
Carbinoxamine
Chlorpheniramine
Clemastine
Dexchlorpheniramine
Diphenhydramine
Diphenylpyraline
Disulfiram
Doxylamine
Ethchlorvynol
Isocarboxazid
Oral contraceptives
Phenelzine
Pheniramine
Pyrilamine
Tranylcypromine
Trichloroethylene
Tripelennamine
Triprolidine

CATARACTS

Alcohol
Amiodarone
Betamethasone
Busulfan
Chloroquine
Chlorpromazine
Chlorprothixene
Cortisone
Deferoxamine
Demecarium
Dexamethasone
Diazoxide
Echothiophate
Edrophonium
Fluphenazine
Haloperidol
Hydrocortisone
Hydroxychloroquine
Isoflurophate
Mesoridazine
Methdilazine
Methylprednisolone
Mitotane
Neostigmine
Perphenazine
Phenmetrazine
Physostigmine
Prednisolone
Prednisone
Prochlorperazine
Promazine
Promethazine
Thiethylperazine
Thioridazine

Thiothixene
Triamcinolone
Trifluoperazine
Trimeprazine

CORNEAL DEPOSITS

Alcohol
Amiodarone
Aurothioglucose
Bismuth subsalicylate
Calcitriol
Chloroquine
Chlorpromazine
Chlorprothixene
Echothiophate
Epinephrine
Ergocalciferol
Ferrous fumarate
Ferrous gluconate
Ferrous sulfate
Fluphenazine
Gold sodium thiomalate
Hydroxychloroquine
Indomethacin
Iron dextran
Mesoridazine
Methdilazine
Perphenazine
Prochlorperazine
Promazine
Promethazine
Quinacrine
Thiethylperazine
Thioridazine
Thiothixene

Trifluoperazine
Trimeprazine
Vitamin D_2/D_3

DECREASED VISION

Acetaminophen
Acetazolamide
Acetohexamide
Alcohol
Allopurinol
Amantadine
Amiodarone
Amitriptyline
Amoxapine
Amphetamine
Amphotericin B
Amyl nitrite
Anisotropine
Antipyrine
Aprobarbital
Aspirin
Atropine
Azatadine
Bacitracin
Baclofen
Belladonna
Bendroflumethiazide
Benzphetamine
Benzthiazide
Benztropine
Betamethasone
Biperiden
Brompheniramine
Bupivacaine
Busulfan

Butabarbital
Butalbital
Capreomycin
Carbamazepine
Carbinoxamine
Carbon dioxide
Carisoprodol
Carmustine
Chloral hydrate
Chlorambucil
Chloramphenicol
Chlorcyclizine
Chlordiazepoxide
Chloroprocaine
Chloroquine
Chlorothiazide
Chlorpheniramine
Chlorpromazine
Chlorpropamide
Chlorprothixene
Chlortetracycline
Chlorthalidone
Clemastine
Clidinium
Clofibrate
Clomiphene
Clonazepam
Clonidine
Clorazepate
Cocaine
Codeine
Colchicine
Cortisone
Cyclizine
Cyclophosphamide

Decreased Vision   *(continued)*
Cycloserine
Cyproheptadine
Dacarbazine
Dantrolene
Dapsone
Deferoxamine
Demecarium
Demeclocycline
Deserpidine
Desipramine
Deslanoside
Dexamethasone
Dexchlorpheniramine
Dextroamphetamine
Dextrothyroxine
Diazepam
Diazoxide
Dibucaine
Dichlorphenamide
Dicumarol
Dicyclomine
Diethylpropion
Digitoxin
Digoxin
Diphenhydramine
Diphenylpyraline
Diphtheria-pertussis-tetanus vaccine adsorbed
Disopyramide
Disulfiram
Doxepin
Doxycycline
Doxylamine
Droperidol
Dyclonine

Echothiophate
Edrophonium
Ephedrine
Epinephrine
Ergotamine
Erythrityl tetranitrate
Ethacrynic acid
Ethambutol
Ethchlorvynol
Ethionamide
Ethosuximide
Etidocaine
Fenfluramine
Floxuridine
Fluorouracil
Fluphenazine
Flurazepam
Furosemide
Gentamicin
Glutethimide
Glycerin
Glycopyrrolate
Griseofulvin
Guanethidine
Haloperidol
Heparin
Hexachlorophene
Hexocyclium
Homatropine
Hydralazine
Hydrochlorothiazide
Hydrocortisone
Hydroflumethiazide
Hydromorphone
Hydroxyamphetamine

Decreased Vision   *(continued)*
Hydroxychloroquine
Ibuprofen
Imipramine
Indomethacin
Influenza virus vaccine
Insulin
Iodide and iodine solution and compounds
Iodochlorhydroxyquin
Iodoquinol
Iron dextran
Isocarboxazid
Isoflurophate
Isoniazid
Isopropamide
Isosorbide
Isosorbide dinitrate
Kanamycin
Ketamine
Ketaprofen
Levodopa
Levothyroxine
Lidocaine
Liothyronine
Liotrix
Lithium carbonate
Lomustine
Lorazepam
Loxapine
Mannitol
Measles virus vaccine (live)
Mecamylamine
Mechlorethamine
Meclizine
Mefenamic acid

Melphalan
Mepenzolate
Meperidine
Mephobarbital
Mepivacaine
Meprobamate
Mesoridazine
Methacycline
Methadone
Methamphetamine
Metharbital
Methazolamide
Methdilazine
Methocarbamol
Methohexital
Methotrexate
Methscopolamine
Methsuximide
Methyclothiazide
Methyl alcohol
Methyldopa
Methylene blue
Methylergonovine
Methylphenidate
Methylprednisolone
Methyprylon
Methysergide
Metoclopramide
Metolazone
Metoprolol
Minocycline
Mitomycin
Mitotane
Morphine
Nalidixic acid

Decreased Vision   *(continued)*
Naloxone
Naphazoline
Naproxen
Neostigmine
Niacin
Niacinamide
Nicotinyl alcohol
Nitrofurantoin
Nitroglycerin
Nortriptyline
Nystatin
Opium
Oral contraceptives
Orphenadrine
Oxazepam
Oxygen
Oxymorphone
Oxytetracycline
Pentaerythritol tetranitrate
Pentazocine
Pentobarbital
Perphenazine
Phendimetrazine
Phenelzine
Phenindione
Pheniramine
Phenmetrazine
Phenobarbital
Phensuximide
Phentermine
Phenylbutazone
Phenylephrine
Phenytoin
Physostigmine

Poliovirus vaccine
Polymyxin B
Polythiazide
Pralidoxime
Prazepam
Prednisolone
Prednisone
Primidone
Procaine
Prochlorperazine
Procyclidine
Promazine
Promethazine
Propantheline
Propoxyphene
Propanolol
Protriptyline
Pyridostigmine
Pyrilamine
Quinacrine
Quinethazone
Quinidine
Quinine
Rabies immune globulin and vaccine
Rauwolfia serpentina
Rescinnamine
Reserpine
Rifampin
Rubella virus vaccine
Scopolamine
Secobarbital
Sildenafil citrate
Sodium salicylate
Spironolactone
Streptomycin

Decreased Vision   *(continued)*
Sulfacetamide
Sulfamethizole
Sulfamethoxazole
Sulfanilamide
Sulfasalazine
Sulfathiazole
Sulfisoxazole
Sulindac
Talbutal
Tamoxifen
Tetracaine
Tetracycline
Tetrahydrozoline
Thiabendazole
Thiamylal
Thiethylperazine
Thioridazine
Thiothixene
Thyroglobulin
Thyroid
Timolol
Tolazamide
Tolbutamide
Tranylcypromine
Triamcinolone
Trichlormethiazide
Tridihexethyl
Trifluoperazine
Trihexyphenidyl
Trimeprazine
Trimethaphan
Trimipramine
Tripelennamine
Triprolidine

Urea
Vinblastine
Warfarin

INCREASED INTRAOCULAR PRESSURE

Atropine
Betamethasone
Carbon dioxide
Cortisone
Demecarium
Dexamethasone
Echothiophate
Homatropine
Hydrocortisone
Insulin
Isoflurophate
Ketamine
Methylprednisolone
Mitomycin
Prednisolone
Prednisone
Scopolamine
Sodium chloride
Succinylcholine
Tolazoline
Triamcinolone
Urokinase

MYASTHENIC NEUROMUSCULAR BLOCKING EFFECT

Bacitracin
Betamethasone
Chlorpromazine
Chlortetracycline
Colistimethate

Myasthenic Neuromuscular Blocking Effect   *(continued)*
Colistin
Cortisone
Demeclocycline
Dexamethasone
Dextrothyroxine
Doxycycline
Fluphenazine
Gentamicin
Hydrocortisone
Kanamycin
Levothyronine
Liothyronine
Liotrix
Lithium carbonate
Mesoridazine
Methacycline
Methdilazine
Methoxyflurane
Methylprednisolone
Minocycline
Neomycin
Oxtetracycline
Paramethadione
Penicillamine
Perphenazine
Phenytoin
Polymyxin B
Prednisolone
Prednisone
Prochlorperazine
Promazine
Promethazine
Propranolol
Quinidine

Streptomycin
Sulfacetamide
Sulfamethizole
Sulfamethoxazole
Sulfanilamide
Sulfasalazine
Sulfathiazole
Sulfisoxazole
Tetracycline
Thiethylperazine
Thioridazine
Thyroglobulin
Thyroid
Timolol
Triamcinolone
Trifluoperazine
Trimeprazine
Trimethadione
Trimethaphan

NYSTAGMUS

Alcohol
Amitriptyline
Amoxapine
Aspirin
Aurothioglucose
Baclofen
Bupivacaine
Butabarbital
Butalbital
Calcitriol
Carbamazepine
Carbinoxamine
Carisoprodol

Nystagmus *(continued)*
Cefazolin
Cephalexin
Cephradine
Chloral hydrate
Chlordiazepoxide
Chloroprocaine
Chloroquine
Chlorpromazine
Clemastine
Clonazepam
Clorazepate
Colistimethate
Colistin
Desipramine
Diazepam
Diphenhydramine
Diphenylpyraline
Disulfiram
Doxepin
Doxylamine
Ergocalciferol
Ethacrynic acid
Ethchlorvynol
Ethotoin
Etidocaine
Fenfluramine
Floxuridine
Fluorouracil
Fluphenazine
Flurazepam
Glutethimide
Gold sodium thiomalate
Hydroxychloroquine
Imipramine

Influenza virus vaccine
Insulin
Iodochlorhydroxyquin
Iodoquinol
Isoniazid
Ketamine
Lidocaine
Lithium carbonate
Lorazepam
Measles virus vaccine
Mephenytoin
Mephobarbital
Mepivacaine
Meprobamate
Mesoridazine
Metaraminol
Metharbital
Methdilazine
Methocarbamol
Methohexital
Methoxamine
Methyl alcohol
Metoclopramide
Metocurine iodide
Nalidixic acid
Nitrofurantoin
Norepinephrine
Nortriptyline
Oxazepam
Paramethadione
Pentazocine
Pentobarbital
Perphenazine
Phenelzine
Phenobarbital

Nystagmus   *(continued)*
Phenytoin
Poliovirus vaccine
Polymyxin B
Prazepam
Primidone
Procaine
Procarbazine
Prochlorperazine
Promazine
Promethazine
Protriptyline
Quinine
Rabies immune globulin and vaccine
Rubella virus vaccine (live)
Secobarbital
Sodium salicylate
Streptomycin
Talbutal
Tetanus toxoid
Thiamylal
Thiethylperazine
Thioridazine
Tranylcypromine
Trifluoperazine
Trimeprazine
Trimethadione
Trimipramine
Tripelennamine
Tubocurarine
Valproic acid
Vitamin A
Vitamin D_2
Vitamin D_3

PAPILLEDEMA SECONDARY TO PSEUDOTUMOR CEREBRI

Betamethasone
Chlortetracycline
Cortisone
Demeclocycline
Dexamethasone
Diphtheria-pertussis-tetanus vaccine adsorbed
Doxycycline
Gentamicin
Griseofulvin
Hydrocortisone
Isotretinoin
Methacycline
Methylprednisolone
Minocycline
Nalidixic acid
Nitrofurantoin
Oral contraceptives
Oxytetracycline
Prednisolone
Prednisone
Tetracycline
Triamcinolone
Vitamin A

PARESIS OF EXTRAOCULAR MUSCLES

Acetohexamide
Alcohol
Amitriptyline
Amphotericin B
Aprobarbital
Aspirin

Paresis of Extraocular Muscles   *(continued)*
Aurothioglucone
Bupivacaine
Butabarbital
Butalbital
Carisoprodol
Chloral hydrate
Chlordiazepoxide
Chloroprocaine
Chloroquine
Chlorpropamide
Clonazepam
Clorazepate
Colchicine
Desipramine
Diazepam
Digitoxin
Diphtheria-pertussis-tetanus vaccine adsorbed
Disulfiram
Ethambutol
Etidocaine
Flurazepam
Gold sodium thiomalate
Hydroxychloroquine
Imipramine
Influenza virus vaccine
Insulin
Isocarboxazid
Isoniazid
Levodopa
Lidocaine
Lorazepam
Measles virus vaccine (live)
Mephobarbital
Mepivacaine

Meprobamate
Metharbital
Methohexital
Methyl alcohol
Methyldopa
Methylene blue
Metoclopramide
Metocurine iodide
Nalidixic acid
Nitrofurantoin
Nortriptyline
Oral contraceptives
Oxazepam
Pentobarbital
Phenelzine
Phenobarbital
Phenylbutazone
Phenytoin
Poliovirus vaccine
Prazepam
Primidone
Procaine
Protriptyline
Quinacrine
Rabies immune globulin and vaccine
Secobarbital
Sodium salicylate
Succinylcholine
Talbutal
Thiamylal
Tolazamide
Tolbutamide
Tranylcypromine
Tubocurarine
Vinblastine

Paresis of Extraocular Muscles   *(continued)*
Vincristine
Vitamin A
Vitamin D_2
Vitamin D_3

RETINAL OR MACULAR PIGMENTARY CHANGES OR DEPOSITS

Azathioprine
Chloramphenicol
Chloroquine
Chlorpromazine
Chlorprothixene
Clofazimine
Ethambutol
Fluphenazine
Hydroxychloroquine
Mesoridazine
Methdilazine
Mitotane
Penicillamine
Perphenazine
Prochlorperazine
Promazine
Promethazine
Quinine
Thiethylperazine
Thioridazine
Thiothixene
Trifluoperazine
Trimeprazine

TOXIC AMBLYOPIA

Alcohol
Amitriptyline

Antipyrine
Aprobarbital
Aspirin
Betamethasone
Butabarbital
Butalbital
Chloramphenicol
Chloroquine
Chlorpromazine
Cortisone
Desipramine
Dexamethasone
Disulfiram
Ethambutol
Ethchlorvynol
Fluphenazine
Hexachlorophene
Hydrocortisone
Hydroxychloroquine
Ibuprofen
Imipramine
Influenza virus vaccine
Iodide and iodine solution and compounds
Iodochlorhydroxyquin
Iodoquinol
Isoniazid
Mephobarbital
Mesoridazine
Metharbital
Methdilazine
Methohexital
Methyl alcohol
Methylprednisolone
Niacin
Niacinamide
Nicotinyl alcohol

Toxic Amblyopia   *(continued)*
Nortriptyline
Pentobarbital
Perphenazine
Phenobarbital
Phenylbutazone
Prednisolone
Prednisone
Primidone
Prochlorperazine
Promazine
Promethazine
Protriptyline
Quinidine
Quinine
Secobarbital
Sodium salicylate
Streptomycin
Talbutal
Thiamylal
Thiethylperazine
Thioridazine
Triamcinolone
Trifluoperazine
Trimeprazine

VISUAL HALLUCINATIONS

Alcohol
Amantadine
Amitriptyline
Amoxapine
Amphetamine
Amyl nitrate
Aprobarbital

Aspirin
Atropine
Azatadine
Baclofen
Belladonna
Benztropine
Biperiden
Bismuth subsalicylate
Brompheniramine
Butabarbital
Butalbital
Calcitriol
Carbamazepine
Carbinoxamine
Carbon dioxide
Cefazolin
Cephalexin
Cephradine
Chloral hydrate
Chlorcyclizine
Chloroquine
Chlorpheniramine
Chlorpromazine
Chlortetracycline
Cimetidine
Clemastine
Clonidine
Cyclizine
Cycloserine
Cyproheptadine
Dantrolene
Demeclocycline
Desipramine
Dexchlorpheniramine
Dextroamphetamine

Visual Hallucinations   *(continued)*
Digoxin
Diphenhydramine
Diphenylpyraline
Disulfiram
Doxepin
Doxycycline
Doxylamine
Droperidol
Ephedrine
Ergocalciferol
Ethchlorvynol
Fluphenazine
Flurazepam
Furosemide
Glutethimide
Glycerin
Griseofulvin
Haloperidol
Homatropine
Hydroxychloroquine
Hydroxyurea
Imipramine
Indomethacin
Iodide and iodine solution and compounds
Isosorbide
Ketamine
Levodopa
Mannitol
Meclizine
Mephobarbital
Mesoridazine
Methacycline
Methamphetamine
Metharbital

Methdilazine
Methohexital
Methscopolamine
Methyldopa
Methylphenidate
Methyprylon
Minocycline
Naloxone
Nortriptyline
Oxytetracycline
Pargyline
Pentazocine
Pentobarbital
Perphenazine
Pheniramine
Phenmetrazine
Phenobarbital
Phenylbutazone
Phenytoin
Primidone
Prochlorperazine
Procyclidine
Promazine
Promethazine
Propranolol
Protriptyline
Pyrilamine
Quinine
Scopolamine
Secobarbital
Sodium salicylate
Sulfacetamide
Sulfamethizole
Sulfamethoxazole
Sulfanilamide

Visual Hallucinations   *(continued)*
Sulfasalazine
Sulfathiazole
Sulfisoxazole
Talbutal
Tetracycline
Thiamylal
Thiethylperazine
Thioridazine
Timolol
Trifluoperazine
Trihexyphenidyl
Trimeprazine
Trimipramine
Tripelennamine
Triprolidine
Urea
Valproic acid
Vitamin D_2
Vitamin D_3

NOTES

18

Insurance and Medicare Codes

DIAGNOSTIC (ICD-9) CODES

Accommodative insufficiency	367.50
Achromatopsia	368.54
Acne rosacea	695.3
After cataract (obscuring vision)	366.53
Amaurosis fugax	362.34
Amblyopia (unspecified)	368.00
Amblyopia, refractive	368.03
Amblyopia, strabismic	368.01
Amblyopia, tobacco	377.34
Angioid streaks	363.43
Angiomatosis, retinal	759.6
Aniridia, congenital	743.45
Aniseikonia	367.32
Anisocoria, of pupil	379.41
Aphakia, acquired	379.31
Aphakia, congenital	743.35
Arcus senilis	371.41
Argyll-Robertson pupil (nonsyphilitic)	379.45
Argyll-Robertson pupil (syphilitic)	094.89
Asteroid hyalitis	379.22
Asthenopia	368.13
Asthenopia, accommodative	367.4
Astigmatism, irregular	367.22

Astigmatism, regular	367.21
Band-shaped keratopathy	371.43
Bitot's spots	264.1
Black eye	921.00
Blepharitis (unspecified)	373.00
Blepharoconjunctivitis	372.20
Blepharospasm	333.81
Blurred vision	368.10
Branch retinal artery occlusion	362.32
Branch retinal vein occlusion	362.36
Bullous keratopathy	371.23
Buphthalmos	743.20
Burn, corneal and conjunctival	940.4
Burn, eyelids	940.1
Burn, of eye(s)(unspecified)	940.9
Canaliculitis, acute	375.31
Canaliculitis, chronic	375.41
Carcinoma, of eyelid	232.1
Cataract, congenital (unspecified)	743.30
Cataract, cortical, senile	366.15
Cataract, immature	366.12
Cataract, mature	366.17
Cataract, nonsenile (unspecified)	366.00
Cataract, nuclear (senile)	366.16
Cataract, secondary (unspecified)	366.50
Cataract, traumatic (unspecified)	366.20
Cataract (unspecified)	366.9
Cellulitis, orbital	376.1
Central retinal artery occlusion	362.31
Central retinal vein occlusion	362.35
Chalazion	373.2
Chorioretinal scar (unspecified)	363.30
Chorioretinitis, disseminated (unspecified)	363.10
Chorioretinitis, focal (unspecified)	363.00
Chorioretinitis (unspecified)	363.20

Choroidal degeneration (unspecified)	363.40
Choroidal detachment	363.70
Choroidal rupture	363.63
Choroideremia	363.55
Choroiditis	363.20
Coats' syndrome	362.12
Cogan's syndrome	370.52
Coloboma, choroid	743.59
Coloboma of eyelid	743.62
Coloboma of iris (congenital)	743.46
Coloboma of optic disc (congenital)	743.57
Coloboma, retinal	743.56
Coloboma, scleral	743.47
Color blindness (acquired)	368.55
Commotio retinae	921.3
Concretion, conjunctival	372.54
Concussion, ocular	921.3
Conjugate gaze, palsy of	378.81
Conjunctival cysts	372.75
Conjunctival deposits	372.56
Conjunctival edema	373.73
Conjunctival hemorrhage	372.72
Conjunctival pigmentation	372.55
Conjunctivitis, acute	372.00
Conjunctivitis, chronic	372.10
Conjunctivitis (unspecified)	372.30
Convergence excess	378.84
Convergence insufficiency	378.83
Corneal abrasion	918.1
Corneal degeneration (unspecified)	371.40
Corneal dystrophy (unspecified)	371.50
Corneal edema	371.20
Corneal lesion	371.42
Corneal foreign body	930.00
Corneal neovascularization	370.60

Corneal opacity (unspecified)	371.00
Corneal ulcer (unspecified)	370.00
Cystoid macular degeneration	362.54
Dacryoadenitis (unspecified)	375.00
Dacryocystitis	375.30
Dacryolith	375.57
Dermatitis, contact	692.9
Descemet's membrane, rupture of	371.33
Deuteranomaly	368.52
Developmental disorder	315.9
Diabetes, with ophthalmic manifestations	250.5
Diabetic retinopathy, background	362.01
Diabetic retinopathy, proliferative	362.02
Diplopia	368.2
Dizziness	780.4
Drusen of optic disc	377.21
Drusen, retinal	362.57
Dry eye syndrome	375.15
Duane's syndrome	378.71
Dyslexia	784.61
Ecchymosis of eye (traumatic)	921.00
Ectopia of pupil	364.75
Ectropion of eyelid	374.10
Elschnig's pearls	366.51
Emphysema of eyelid	374.85
Emphysema, orbital	376.89
Endophthalmitis	360.00
Enlarged blind spot, visual field	368.42
Endophthalmos (unspecified)	376.50
Entropion of eyelid	374.00
Epicanthus of eyelid (congenital)	743.63
Epiphora	375.20
Episcleritis	379.00
Esophoria	378.41
Esotropia	378.00

Exophoria	378.42
Exophthalmos	376.30
Exotropia	378.10
Foreign body, conjunctival	930.1
Foreign body, corneal	930.00
Foreign body, intraocular, magnetic (new)	871.5
Foreign body, intraocular, magnetic (old)	360.50
Foreign body, intraocular, nonmagnetic (new)	871.6
Foreign body, intraocular, nonmagnetic (old)	360.60
Fundus flavimaculatus	362.76
Glaucoma, chronic, open-angle	365.11
Glaucoma, congenital	743.20
Glaucoma, corticosteroid-induced	365.31
Glaucoma, low-tension	365.12
Glaucoma, narrow-angle (unspecified)	365.20
Glaucoma, open-angle	365.10
Glaucoma, phacolytic	365.51
Glaucoma, pigmentary	365.13
Glaucoma, pseudoexfoliation	365.52
Glaucoma, suspected	365.00
Glaucoma (unspecified)	365.9
Headache	784.00
Hemangioma, choroidal	228.09
Hemangioma, retinal	228.03
Hemangioma (unspecified site)	228.00
Hemianopsia, homonymous	368.46
Hemianopsia, bitemporal	368.47
Herpes simplex (with ophthalmic complications)	054.40
Herpes zoster (with ophthalmic complications)	053.20
Histoplasmosis, ocular	115.02
Hollenhorst plaque	362.33
Hordeolum, external	373.11
Hordeolum, internal	373.12
Hyperopia	367.00
Hyperphoria	378.43

Hypertension	401.9
Hypertropia	378.31
Hyphema	364.41
Hypopyon	364.05
Hypotony, of eye	360.30
Hysterical blindness	300.11
Injury of eye	921.9
Iridis, rubeosis	364.42
Iridocyclitis (acute and subacute)	364.00
Iridocyclitis (chronic, unspecified)	364.10
Iridodialysis	364.76
Iridodonesis	364.8
Iridoplegia	379.49
Iris, adhesions of	364.70
Iris, atrophy of	364.51
Iritis, acute	364.00
Iritis, chronic	364.10
Keratitis, superficial	370.20
Keratoconjunctivitis	370.40
Keratoconus	371.60
Keratoglobus	371.70
Krukenberg's spindle	371.13
Laceration of eyeball	871.4
Laceration of eyelid	870.8
Lacrimal duct obstruction (neonatal)	375.55
Lacrimal duct stenosis (acquired)	375.56
Lacrimal punctum stenosis	375.52
Lacrimal sac stenosis	375.54
Lagophthalmos of eyelid	374.20
Learning difficulties	315.2
Lens subluxation	379.32
Lymphoma, benign	229.00
Lymphoma, malignant	202.8
Macular cyst	362.54
Macular degeneration, dry (nonexudative)	362.51

Macular degeneration, senile (unspecified)	362.50
Macular degeneration, wet (exudative)	362.52
Macular hole	362.54
Macular puckering	362.56
Macular scars	363.32
Maculopathy, toxic	362.55
Madarosis of eyelid	374.55
Malingerer	V65.2
Marcus Gunn syndrome	742.8
Medullated nerve fibers	743.57
Meibomitis	373.12
Melanoma, choroidal	190.6
Melanoma of eyelid (malignant)	172.1
Melanoma, retinal	190.5
Melanosis, conjunctival	372.55
Melanosis, scleral	379.19
Metamorphopsia	368.14
Microaneurysm, retinal	362.14
Molluscum contagiosum	078.0
Monofixation syndrome	378.34
Muscae volitantes	379.24
Myasthenia gravis	358.0
Myopia	367.1
Myopia, progressive	360.21
Nasolacrimal duct obstruction	375.56
Nearsightedness	367.1
Neoplasm of eye (benign)	224.9
Neoplasm of eye (malignant)	190.9
Neovascularization, choroidal	362.16
Neovascularization, corneal	370.60
Neovascularization of iris	364.42
Neovascularization, retinal	362.16
Neuroretinitis	363.05
Night blindness	368.60
Normal state	V65.5

Nystagmus	379.50
Ocular hypertension	365.04
Oculomotor dysfunction	378.9
Oculomotor paralysis	344.8
Ophthalmoplegia (total)	378.56
Optic atrophy	377.10
Optic chiasm, disorders of	377.5
Optic neuritis	377.30
Optic neuritis, meningococcal	036.81
Optic neuropathy, ischemic	377.34
Optic neuropathy, nutritional	377.33
Optic neuropathy, toxic	377.34
Pain of eye	379.91
Pannus, corneal	370.62
Panuveitis	360.12
Papilledema	377.00
Papillitis	377.31
Papilloma	078.1
Paresis, accommodation	367.51
Paresis of eye muscle	378.55
Pars planitis	363.21
Photophobia	368.13
Photopsia	368.15
Phthisis bulbi	360.41
Pinguecula	372.51
Posterior staphyloma	379.12
Posterior synechia	364.71
Presbyopia	367.4
Protanomaly	368.51
Pseudopapilledema	377.24
Pseudoretinitis pigmentosa	362.65
Pterygium	372.40
Ptosis	374.30
Recurrent corneal erosion	371.42
Retinal degeneration, peripheral	362.60

Retinal detachment, serous	361.2
Retinal detachment, traction	361.81
Retinal detachment (unspecified)	361.9
Retinal dystrophy, hereditary (unspecified)	362.70
Retinal edema	362.83
Retinal hemorrhage	362.81
Retinal microaneurysms	362.14
Retinal neovascularization	362.16
Retinal tear with detachment	361.00
Retinal tear without detachment	361.30
Retinal vascular occlusion	362.30
Retinal vasculitis	362.18
Retinitis	363.20
Retinitis pigmentosa	362.74
Retinoblastoma	190.5
Retinochoroiditis	363.20
Retinoschisis	361.10
Retrobulbar optic neuritis	377.32
Rubeosis iridis	364.42
Scleritis	379.00
Scotoma, central	368.41
Stargardt's disease	362.75
Strabismus, concomitant	378.30
Strabismus, paralytic	378.50
Stye, external	373.11
Stye, internal	373.12
Subluxation of lens	379.32
Synchysis scintillans	379.22
Tortuous retinal vessel, congenital	747.6
Toxoplasmosis, chorioretinitis	130.2
Trachoma	076.9
Transient blindness	368.12
Trichiasis of eyelid	374.05
Tritanomaly	368.53
Ulcer, corneal	370.00

Uveitis, anterior	364.3
Uveitis, posterior	363.20
Verruca	078.1
Vision, loss of (both eyes)	369.3
Vision, loss of (one eye)	369.8
Visual disturbances, subjective (unspecified)	368.10
Visual field defect	368.40
Vitreous degeneration	379.21
Vitreous detachment	379.21
Vitreous hemorrhage	379.23
Vitreous floaters	379.24
Vitreous prolapse	379.26
Vogt-Koyanagi syndrome	364.24
Warts, viral	078.1
Xanthelasma of eyelid	374.51

EVALUATION AND MANAGEMENT CODING

Determining the correct evaluation and management (E/M) code for a patient encounter requires three steps: (1) level of history, (2) level of examination, and (3) level of decision making.

Determining the Correct Code for a New Patient Office Visit*

	Level I 99201	Level II 99202	Level III 99203	Level IV 99204	Level V 99205
History	Problem focused	Expanded problem focused	Detailed	Comprehensive	Comprehensive
Examination	Problem focused	Expanded problem focused	Detailed	Comprehensive	Comprehensive
Decision making	Straight-forward	Straight-forward	Low complexity	Moderate complexity	High complexity

*To select the correct code, draw a line up the column with three circles. Otherwise, draw a line up the column with the circle nearest the left.

Determining the Correct Code for an Established Patient Office Visit*

	Level I 99211	Level II 99212	Level III 99213	Level IV 99214	Level V 99215
History	—	Problem focused	Expanded problem focused	Detailed	Comprehensive
Examination	—	Problem focused	Expanded problem focused	Detailed	Comprehensive
Decision making	—	Straightforward	Low complexity	Moderate complexity	High complexity

*To select the correct code, draw a line up the column with two or three circles. Otherwise, draw a line up the column with the circle second from the right.

Determining the Correct Code for an Office or Other Outpatient Consultation for a New or Established Patient*

	Level I 99201	Level II 99202	Level III 99203	Level IV 99204	Level V 99205
History	Problem focused	Expanded problem focused	Detailed	Comprehensive	Comprehensive
Examination	Problem focused	Expanded problem focused	Detailed comprehensive	Comprehensive	
Decision making	Straightforward	Straightforward	Low complexity	Moderate complexity	High complexity

*To select the correct code, draw a line up the column with three circles. Otherwise, draw a line up the column with the circle nearest the left.

Step 1: Documentation of History*

History of Present Illness (HPI)	Review of Systems (ROS)	Past Family and Social History (PFSH)	Type of History
Brief	None	None	**Problem focused**
Brief	Problem pertinent	None	**Expanded problem focused**
Extended	Extended	Pertinent	**Detailed**
Extended	Complete	Complete	**Comprehensive**

*Each of the three elements (HPI, ROS, PFSH) must be met. A chief complaint is necessary. Draw a line across a row with three circles to determine the type of history. Otherwise, draw a line across the row with a circle closest to the top.

History of Present Illness

The history of present illness (HPI) may include the following elements:

- Location
- Timing
- Quality
- Context
- Severity
- Modifying factors
- Duration
- Associated signs and symptoms

Brief = 1 to 3 elements.
Extended = 4 or more elements, or the status of at least three chronic inactive conditions.

Review of Systems

The following systems are recognized for review of systems (ROS):

- Constitutional symptoms
- Eyes
- Ears, nose, and throat

- Cardiovascular
- Respiratory
- Gastrointestinal
- Genitourinary
- Musculoskeletal
- Integumentary (skin/breast)
- Neurologic
- Psychiatric
- Endocrine
- Hematologic, lymphatic
- Allergic/immunologic

Problem pertinent = 1 system reviewed.
Extended = 2–9 systems reviewed.
Complete = 10 or more systems reviewed.

Past Family and Social History

There are three areas of the past family and social history (PFSH):

- Past history: A review of current medical conditions, prior illnesses and injuries, operations, hospitalizations, allergies, and immunization status.
- Family history: Information about the health status or cause of death of parents, siblings, and children. Specific diseases related to problems in the chief complaint, HPI, or ROS.
- Social history: An age-appropriate review of significant activities that may include such information as marital status; living arrangement; occupational history; use of drugs, alcohol, and tobacco; extent of education, and sexual activity.

Pertinent = at least one specific item from one area.
Complete for established patient office visit = at least one specific item from two areas.
Complete for new patient office visit and consultations = one specific item from each of the three areas.

Step 2: Documentation of an Eye Examination*

Type of Examination	Required Number of Elements
Problem focused	One or more
Expanded problem focused	At least six
Detailed	At least nine
Comprehensive	All eye elements plus one neurologic/psychiatric element

*All components of each element must be examined. At least one component must be documented. Describe abnormal findings and relevant negatives. Clear or normal is acceptable.

Components of eye examination and neurologic/psychiatric examination

Eye	Ocular motility including primary gaze alignment
	Inspection of bulbar and palpebral conjunctivae
	Examination of ocular adnexae including lids, lacrimal gland, lacrimal drainage, orbits, and preauricular lymph nodes
	Examination of pupils and irides including shape, size, reaction, and morphology
	Slit-lamp examination of corneas including epithelium, stroma, endothelium, and tear film
	Slit-lamp examination of the anterior chambers including depth, cells, and flare
	Slit-lamp examination of the lenses including clarity, anterior and posterior capsule, cortex, and nucleus
	Measurement of intraocular pressures (except in children and patients with trauma or infectious disease)
	Ophthalmoscopic examination through dilated pupils (unless contraindicated) of:
	Optic discs including size, cup-to-disc ratio, appearance, and nerve fiber layer
	Posterior segments including retina and vessels
Neurologic/ psychiatric	Brief assessment of mental status including:
	Orientation to time, place, and person
	Mood and affect

Step 3: Determining the Level of Decision Making*

Number of diagnoses or management options	≤1 minimal	2 limited	3 multiple	≥4 extensive
Amount and complexity of data	≤1 minimal	2 limited	3 moderate	≥4 extensive
Overall risk	1 minimal	2 low	3 moderate	4 high
Type of decision making	**Straight-forward**	**Low complexity**	**Moderate complexity**	**High complexity**

*To select the correct level of decision making, draw a line down any column with two or three circles. Otherwise, draw a line down the column with the second circle from the left.

Number of Diagnoses or Management Options Considered

Self limited/minor problem	= 1 point
Established/stable problem	= 1 point
Established/worsening problem	= 2 points
New problem—no additional workup	= 3 points
New problem—needs additional workup	= 4 points
Total points	_____

Amount and Complexity of Diagnostic Tests

Review and/or order clinical lab tests	= 1 point
Review and/or order radiology tests	= 1 point
Review and/or order medical tests	= 1 point
Discuss test results with performing doctor	= 1 point
Independent review of image, tracing, or specimen	= 2 points
Decision to obtain records/history from third party	= 1 point
Review and summarization of record/history	= 2 points
Total points	_____

Determining the Overall Risk*

Level of Risk	Presenting Problem	Diagnostic Procedures Ordered	Management Options Selected
1: Minimal	One self-limited or minor problem	Laboratory tests requiring venipuncture Chest x-rays Schirmer test Electrocardiogram Color vision Visual fields Tonometry Topical diagnostic agents (rose bengal, fluorescein) Potential acuity meter procedure Contrast sensitivity Ultrasound	Rest Superficial dressings
2: Low	Two or more self-limited or minor problems	Physiologic tests not under stress (e.g., glaucoma provocative tests)	Over-the-counter drugs
	One stable chronic illness (e.g., well-controlled glaucoma)	Noncardiovascular imaging studies with contrast (e.g., MRI)	Minor surgery with no identified risk factors
	Acute uncomplicated illness or injury	Superficial needle biopsies Oral fluorescein angioscopy Conjunctival culture Gonioscopy Ophthalmodynamometry	Occlusion Pressure patch

3: Moderate	One or more chronic illnesses with mild exacerbation	Physiologic tests under stress	Minor surgery with identified risk factors
	Two or more chronic illnesses	Deep needle or incisional biopsy	Referral for or decision to perform elective major surgery with no identified risk factors
	Undiagnosed new problem with uncertain prognosis	Retrobulbar injection	Prescription drug management
	Acute illness with multiple symptoms	IV fluorescein angiogram	Therapeutic nuclear medicine
	Acute complicated injury	Corneal culture	
4: High	One or more chronic illnesses with severe exacerbation	Vitreous tap	Elective major surgery with identified risk factors
	Acute or chronic illnesses or injuries that pose a threat to life or bodily function (e.g., multiple trauma, endophthalmitis, retinoblastoma, amaurosis fugax, malignancies of adnexa, angle closure glaucoma)	Anterior chamber tap Fine needle biopsy— orbital ocular	Referral for or decision to perform emergency major surgery Multiple drug therapy requiring intensive monitoring for toxicity

*Circle the highest level of risk in any one category to determine overall risk.

DOCUMENTATION OF AN ENCOUNTER
DOMINATED BY COUNSELING
OR COORDINATION OF CARE

When counseling and/or coordination of care dominates (i.e., is more than 50% of) the physician-patient or family encounter, time becomes the key or controlling factor in qualifying for a particular level of E/M services.

If the physician elects to report the level of service based on counseling and/or coordination of care, the total length of time of the encounter (face-to-face or floor time, as appropriate) should be documented, and the record should describe the counseling and/or activities for coordinating care.

10 minutes	99201
20 minutes	99202
30 minutes	99203
45 minutes	99204
60 minutes	99205

Typical total physician face-to-face time with established patient:

5 minutes	99211
10 minutes	99212
15 minutes	99213
25 minutes	99214
40 minutes	99215

Typical total physician face-to-face time with office or other outpatient consultations:

15 minutes	99241
30 minutes	99242
40 minutes	99243
60 minutes	99244
80 minutes	99245

PROCEDURAL (CPT-4) CODES

Office Services

99201	Problem-focused examination-10 (new patient)
99202	Expanded problem-20 (new patient)
99203	Detailed examination-30 (new patient)
99204	Comprehensive moderately complex-45 (new patient)
99205	Comprehensive complex-60 (new patient)
99211	Service-5 (established patient)
99212	Problem-focused examination-10 (established patient)
99213	Expanded problem-15 (established patient)
99214	Comprehensive moderately complex-25 (established patient)
99215	Highly complex-40 (established patient)
90000	Brief service (new patient)
90010	Limited service (new patient)
92002	Intermediate service (new patient)
92004	Comprehensive service (new patient)
90017	Extended service (new patient)
90030	Minimal service (established patient)
90040	Brief service (established patient)
90050	Limited service (established patient)
92012	Intermediate service (established patient)
92014	Comprehensive service (established patient)
90070	Extended service (established patient)

Home Medical Services

90100	Brief service (new patient)
90110	Limited service (new patient)
90115	Intermediate service (new patient)
90117	Extended service (new patient)
90130	Minimal service (established patient)
90140	Brief service (established patient)
90150	Limited service (established patient)

90160	Intermediate service (established patient)
90170	Extended service (established patient)

Hospital Medical Services

90200	Brief service
90215	Intermediate service
90220	Comprehensive service

Subsequent Hospital Care

90240	Brief service
90250	Limited service
90260	Intermediate service
90270	Extended service
90280	Comprehensive service

Skilled Nursing, Intermediate Care, and Long-Term Care Facilities

90300	Brief service
90315	Intermediate service
90320	Comprehensive service

Subsequent Care

90340	Brief service
90350	Limited service
90360	Intermediate service
90370	Extended service

Nursing Home/Custodial Care Medical Services

90400	Brief service (new patient)
90410	Limited service (new patient)
90415	Intermediate service (new patient)
90420	Comprehensive service (new patient)

90430	Minimal service (established patient)
90440	Brief service (established patient)
90450	Limited service (established patient)
90460	Intermediate service (established patient)
90470	Extended service (established patient)

Consultations

90600	Limited consultation
90605	Intermediate consultation
90610	Extensive consultation
90620	Comprehensive consultation
90630	Complex consultation

Diagnostic Procedures

92018	Initial ophthalmologic examination and evaluation under general anesthesia
92019	Subsequent ophthalmologic examination and evaluation under general anesthesia
92020	Gonioscopy

Visual Fields

92081	Visual field examination with medical diagnostic evaluation; tangent screen autoplot or equivalent (screening)
92082	Quantitative perimetry, e.g., several isopters on Goldmann's perimeter, or equivalent (intermediate)
92083	Static and kinetic perimetry, or equivalent (diagnostic)

Tonometry/Tonography

| 92100 | Serial tonometry |
| 92120 | Tonography with medical diagnostic evaluation, recording indentation tonometry method or perilimbal suction method |

92130   Tonography with water provocation
92140   Provocative tests for glaucoma, with medical diagnostic
         evaluation

Ophthalmoscopy

92225   Extended ophthalmoscopy
92235   Fluorescein angiography
92250   Fundus photography
92260   Ophthalmodynamometry

Ophthalmic Ultrasound Services

76516   A-scan, ultrasonic biometry
76517   B-scan
76519   A-scan with intraocular lens power calculation
76529   Ophthalmic ultrasonic foreign body localization

Other Specialized Services

92283   Color vision examination, extended—e.g., anomaloscope
         or equivalent (not color vision testing with
         pseudoisochromatic plates)
92285   External ocular photography
92534   Optokinetic nystagmus

Microbiology Services

87040   Culture: bacterial, definitive, aerobic; blood (may include
         anaerobic screen)
87070   Any other source
87075   Culture: bacterial, any source; anaerobic (isolation)

Unlisted Diagnostic Procedures

92499   Unlisted diagnostic procedure

Ophthalmic Treatment Services

92340	Monofocal treatment with spectacles, except for aphakia
92341	Bifocal treatment with spectacles, except for aphakia
92342	Multifocal, or other than bifocal, treatment with spectacles, except for aphakia
92352	Monofocal treatment with spectacles for aphakia
92353	Multifocal treatment with spectacles for aphakia
92358	Prosthesis service for aphakia, temporary
92370	Repair and adjustment of spectacles, except for aphakia
92371	Spectacle prosthesis for aphakia

Contact Lens Treatment Services

92070	Prescription and management of contact lens for treatment of disease, including lens supply
92310	Prescription and management of corneal contact lens, for both eyes, except for aphakia
92311	Corneal lens for aphakia, one eye
92312	Corneal lens for aphakia, two eyes
92314	Prescription and management of corneal contact lens by independent technician with optometric supervision, for both eyes, except for aphakia
92315	Corneal lens for aphakia, one eye
92316	Corneal lens for aphakia, two eyes
92325	Modification of contact lens
92326	Replacement of contact lens

Low-Vision Treatment Services

92354	Treatment with spectacle-mounted low-vision aid; single-element system
92355	Telescopic or other compound lens

Vision Therapy Services

90775	Administation and interpretation of developmental tests

92060	Sensorimotor examination with diagnostic evaluation
92065	Orthoptic and/or pleoptic training
95882	Assessment of higher cerebral function with interpretation; cognitive testing and other testing
95999	Unlisted neurologic or neuromuscular diagnostic procedure
98313	Amblyopia diagnostic examination
98314	Binocular vision diagnostic examination—strabismus
98315	Binocular vision diagnostic examination—nonstrabismus
98316	Oculomotor diagnostic examination
98317	Vision development diagnostic examination
98318	Vision perception diagnostic examination
98304	Vision therapy and orthoptics progress examination or office visit
98681	Amblyopia therapy
98682	Binocular vision therapy—strabismus
98683	Binocular therapy—nonstrabismus
98684	Vision development therapy
98685	Oculomotor therapy
98686	Vision perception therapy

Prosthetic Eye Service

| 92330 | Prescription, fitting, and supply of ocular prosthesis (artificial eye) |
| 92335 | Prescription of ocular prosthesis (artificial eye) and direction of fitting and supply by an independent technician |

Special and Administrative Services and Reports

99000	Collection, handling, and/or conveyance of specimen for transfer from the doctor's office to a laboratory
99001	Collection, handling, and/or conveyance of specimen for transfer from the patient's home to a laboratory
99001	Collection, handling, conveyance, and/or other services in connection with the implementation of an order involving devices (e.g., designing, fitting, packaging, handling,

	delivery, mailing)
99012	Telephone calls, phone consultations, or repeated or lengthy phone calls
99050	Services requested after office hours in addition to basic service
99054	Service requested on Sundays and holidays in addition to basic service
99056	Services provided at the request of the patient in a location other than optometrist's office
99058	Office services provided on an emergency basis
99070	Supplies and materials (nonophthalmic) provided by the doctor over and above those usually included with the office visit or other services rendered
99071	Educational supplies, such as books, tapes, and pamphlets, provided by the doctor for the patient's education at cost to doctor
99075	Medical testimony
99080	Special reports such as insurance forms, or the review of medical data to clarify a patient's status—more than the information conveyed in the usual medical communication or standard reporting form
99082	Analysis of information data stored in computers

Surgery

65205	Removal of foreign body, external eye; conjunctival superficial
65210	Conjunctival embedded (includes concretions), subconjunctival, or scleral nonperforating
65220	Corneal foreign body removal, without slit-lamp
65222	Corneal foreign body removal, with slit-lamp
65270	Repair laceration; conjunctival, with or without nonperforating lacerating sclera, direct closure
65275	Repair laceration of cornea, nonperforating, with or without removal of foreign body

| 65280 | Repair laceration of cornea and/or sclera, perforating, not involving uveal tissue |

Cornea

65400	Excision lesion cornea (keratectomy, lamellar, partial), except pterygium
65410	Biopsy cornea
65420	Excision or transposition pterygium; without graft
65430	Scraping cornea, diagnostic, for smear and/or culture
65435	Removal of corneal epithelium; with or without chemocauterization (abrasion, curettage)
65450	Destruction of lesion of cornea by cryotherapy, photocoagulation, or thermocauterization
65710	Keratoplasty (corneal transplant) lamellar; autograft

Anterior Chamber

65800	Paracentesis of anterior chamber eye (separate procedure); with diagnostic aspiration of aqueous
65855	Trabeculoplasty by laser surgery, one or more sessions (defined treatment series)
65865	Severing adhesions in anterior segment of eye, incisional technique (with or without injection air or liquid) (separate procedure); goniosynechiae

Anterior Sclera

66130	Excision of lesion sclera
66150	Fistulization of sclera for glaucoma; trephination with iridectomy
66500	Iridotomy by stab incision (separate procedure); except transfixion
66600	Iridectomy, with corneoscleral or corneal section; for removal of lesion

Lens

| 66821 | Laser surgery (one or more stages) |

66850	Phacofragmentation technique (mechanical or ultrasonic—e.g., phacoemulsification), with aspiration
66984	Extracapsular cataract removal with insertion of intraocular lens prosthesis (one-stage procedure)
66985	Insertion of intraocular lens subsequent to cataract removal (separate procedure)

Retina

67145	Photocoagulation, retinal break
67210	Photocoagulation, localized lesion
67228	Photocoagulation, panretinal

Extraocular Muscles

67311	Strabismus surgery on patient not previously operated on, any procedure, any muscle (may include minor displacement—e.g., for A or V pattern); one muscle
67320	Transposition extraocular muscle (e.g., for paretic muscle), one or more stages, one or more muscles, with displacement of plane of action more than 5 mm

Eyelids

67800	Excision of chalazion, single
67801	Excision of chalazion, multiple, same lid
67820	Correction of trichiasis; epilation, forceps only
67825	Epilation (e.g., by electrosurgery or cryotherapy)
67850	Destruction of lesion of lid margin (up to 1 cm)
67938	Removal of embedded foreign body, eyelid

Conjunctiva

68020	Incision of conjunctiva, drainage of cyst
68135	Destruction of lesion conjunctiva
68200	Subconjunctival injection

Lacrimal System

68760	Closure of lacrimal punctum, thermocauterization

68800	Dilation of lacrimal punctum, with or without irrigation, unilateral or bilateral
68820	Probing of nasolacrimal duct, with or without irrigation, unilateral or bilateral
68830	With insertion of tube or stent (without general anesthesia)
68840	Probing of lacrimal canaliculi, with or without irrigation

Modifiers

#22 Unusual Services: When the service(s) provided is greater than normally required for the listed procedure, it may be identified by adding the modifier 22 to the usual procedure number or by using the separate five-digit modifier code 09922. A report may also be appropriate.

#52 Reduced Services: Under certain circumstances a service or procedure is partially reduced or eliminated at the physician's election. Under these circumstances the service provided can be identified by its usual procedure number and by the addition of the modifier 52, signifying that the service is reduced. This provides a means of reporting reduced services without disturbing the identification of the basic service. The modifier code 09952 may be used as an alternative to modifier 52.

#54 Surgical Care Only: When one physician performs a surgical procedure and another provides preoperative and/or postoperative management, surgical services may be identified by adding the modifier 54 to the usual procedure number or by using the separate five-digit modifier 09954.

#55 Postoperative Management Only: When one physician performs the postoperative management and another physician performs the surgical procedure, the postoperative component may be identified by adding the modifier 55 to the usual procedure number or by using the separate five-digit modifier code 09955.

#75 Concurrent Care, Services Rendered by More Than One Physician: When the patient's condition requires the additional services of more than one physician, each physician may identify his or her services by adding the modifier 75 to the basic service or the service may be reported by using the five-digit modifier code 09975.

#76 Repeat Procedure by Same Physician: The physician may need to indicate that a procedure or service was repeated subsequent to the original service. This circumstance may be reported by adding the modifier 76, or the five-digit modifier code 09976 may be used.

#77 Repeat Procedure by Another Physician: The physician may need to indicate that a basic procedure performed by another physician had to be repeated. This situation may be reported by adding the modifier 77 to the repeated service or by using the separate five-digit modifier code 09977.

NOTES

19

Ocular Syndromes

AICARDI'S SYNDROME

Microphthalmia, retinal lacunae, infantile spasms, seizures, hypotonia, and defects of the corpus colosum.

ALBINISM

Marked deficiency of pigment in iris and choroid, transillumination defects of the iris, decreased visual acuity, nystagmus, myopic astigmatism, photophobia, and macular hypoplasia.

ANIRIDIA

See Chapter 9.

ALBRIGHT'S SYNDROME

Fibrous dysplasia of bones, precocious puberty in females, hearing loss, seizures, mental retardation, proptosis, optic disc edema, and optic atrophy.

ALPORT'S SYNDROME

Autosomal dominant disorder, hemorrhagic nephritis, progressive deafness, anterior lenticonus, and cataracts.

ATAXIA-TELANGIECTASIA

Conjunctival telangiectasia, progressive cerebellar ataxia, nystagmus dysarthria, mental and growth retardation, coarse hair and skin, immunologic deficiency, and pulmonary infections.

AXENFELD'S ANOMALY

Posterior embryotoxin and iris processes to Schwalbe's line.

AXENFELD'S SYNDROME

Axenfeld's anomaly plus glaucoma.

BASAL CELL NEVUS SYNDROME

Tumors of skin and sinuses.

BASSEN-KORNZWEIG SYNDROME

Inability to absorb and transport lipids, atypical retinitis pigmentosa, ptosis, and regressive external ophthalmoplegia (see Chapter 14).

BEHÇET'S SYNDROME

Recurrent uveitis, hypopyon, thrombophlebitis, optic neuritis, aphthous ulcers of the mucous membranes of the mouth and genitalia, skin lesions, and recurrent fever.

BLEPHAROPHIMOSIS SYNDROME

Blepharophimosis (shortened length of palpebral aperture), ptosis, telecanthus, and epicanthus inversus.

CANCER-ASSOCIATED RETINOPATHY SYNDROME

Progressive retinal degeneration and vision loss in cancer patients with antiretinal antibodies.

CHÉDIAK-HIGASHI SYNDROME

Oculocutaneous albinism, anemia, neutropenia, thrombocytopenia, and recurrent infections.

CYSTINURIA

Pigmentary retinopathy and excretion of cystine and other amino acids in the urine.

DE MORSIER'S SYNDROME

Bilateral optic nerve hypoplasia, absent septum pellucidum, and possible pituitary, anomalies including growth deficiency.

DOWN'S SYNDROME

Mental retardation, heart anomalies, hypertelorism, epicanthus, esotropia, myopia, Brushfield (iris) spots, cataracts, and keratoconus.

EDWARDS'S SYNDROME

Trisomy 18: Low birth weight, growth failure, mental retardation, narrow bifrontal diameter, protruding occiput, micrognathia, misshapen ears, finger deformities, atrial and ventricular septal defects, and inguinal and ventral hernias.

FETAL ALCOHOL SYNDROME

Peter's anomaly, telecanthus, and optic nerve hypoplasia.

GOLDENHAR'S SYNDROME

Epibulbar dermoids, facial and midline clefts, vertebral anomalies, and auricular skin appendages.

HERMANSKY-PUDLAK SYNDROME

Oculocutaneous albinism and hemorrhagic diathesis due to defective platelet function.

HOMOCYSTINURIA

Disorder of amino acid metabolism, mental retardation, arachnodactyly, thromboembolism, subluxated lens, spherophakia, cataract, high myopia, and pupillary block glaucoma.

IRIS-NEVUS SYNDROME

Ectopic corneal endothelium grows over the trabecular meshwork and iris, glaucoma, corneal edema, peripheral anterior synechiae, and ectropion uveae.

KEARNS-SAYRE SYNDROME

Heart block, progressive external ophthalmoplegia, and pigmentary retinal degeneration.

LAURENCE-MOON-BARDET-BIEDL SYNDROME

Retinitis pigmentosa, strabismus, microphthalmia, obesity, hypogonadism, short stature, mental retardation, and congenital heart disease.

LOWE'S SYNDROME

X-linked, neuromuscular hypotonia, congenital cataract, glaucoma, and aberration in amino acid metabolism.

MARFAN'S SYNDROME

Subluxed lens; spherophakia; arachnodactyly; tall, lean habitus; and aortic anomalies.

MILLARD-GUBLER SYNDROME

Ipsilateral sixth and seventh nerve palsies with contralateral hemiplegia from lesion at the base of the pons.

MÖBIUS II SYNDROME

Congenital sixth and seventh nerve paralysis, ptosis, facial diplegia, and deafness.

NEUROFIBROMATOSIS

Neurofibromas of lid and orbit, Lisch nodules of iris, retinal glial hamartomas, glaucoma, optic nerve glioma, pulsating exophthalmos from absent sphenoid, and café au lait spots.

OLIVO-PONTO-CEREBELLAR ATROPHY

Retinal degeneration, progressive external ophthalmoplegia, and ataxia.

PARINAUD'S SYNDROME

Most commonly associated with pineal tumor, eyelid retraction, paralysis of upgaze, convergence retraction nystagmus, and light-near dissociation of pupils.

PATAU'S SYNDROME (TRISOMY 13)

Shallow orbital ridge, absent eyebrows, epicanthal folds, microphthalmia, cloudy cornea, cataract, uveal colobomas, intraocular cartilage, persistent hyperplastic primary vitreous, optic nerve hypoplasia, anterior cleavage syndrome, cyclopia, hypertelorism, rocker bottom feet, heart disorders, central nervous system anomalies, cleft lip and palate, deafness, polydactyly, and clenched fist.

PETER'S ANOMALY

Central defect in Descemet's membrane, corneal opacity, iris strands to edge of corneal defect, keratolenticular stalk, and cataracts.

PIERRE-ROBIN SYNDROME

Micrognathia, cleft palate, glossoptosis, microphthalmia, ptosis, myopia, glaucoma, blue sclera, and esotropia.

PURTSCHER'S SYNDROME

Retinal and preretinal hemorrhages, nerve fiber layer infarcts, venous engorgement, and optic nerve edema. Seen most commonly after trauma associated with fractures and in pancreatitis.

REFSUM'S SYNDROME

Phytanic acid storage disease, retinitis pigmentosa, progressive external ophthalmoplegia, spinocerebellar ataxia, deafness, central nervous system degeneration, wasting of extremities, and heart block.

RIEGER'S ANOMALY

Posterior embryotoxin, iris strands, hypoplasia of iris stroma, and corectopia (displaced pupil).

RIEGER'S SYNDROME

Reiger's anomaly plus facial anomalies (maxillary hypoplasia, hypertelorism, hypodontia, oligodontia) and umbilicus.

RUBELLA SYNDROME (CONGENITAL)

Pearly white nuclear lens opacities, salt and pepper fundus, glaucoma, deafness, and cardiac anomalies.

STEELE-RICHARDSON-OLSZEWSKI SYNDROME (PROGRESSIVE SUPRANUCLEAR PALSY)

Pseudobulbar palsy, dysarthria, dystonia, supranuclear ophthalmo-plegia affecting primarily vertical gaze, and dementia.

STICKLER'S SYNDROME

Autosomal dominant, myopia, vitreous liquefaction, radial lattice, retinoschisis, retinal detachment, avascular retinal membranes, glaucoma, cataracts, Pierre-Robin malformation, skeletal abnormalities, and arthritis.

STURGE-WEBER SYNDROME

Vascular port-wine nevus, intracranial angiomas, seizure disorders, secondary glaucomas, and choroidal hemangiomas.

TERSON'S SYNDROME

Intraocular hemorrhages from subarachnoid bleed (as in ruptured aneurysm).

TOLOSA-HUNT SYNDROME

See Orbital Inflammatory Syndrome in Chapter 4.

TUBEROUS SCLEROSIS

Autosomal dominant disorder, facial angiofibromas, "ash leaf" spots of skin, cerebral glial hamartomas, retinal glial hamartomas, and seizures.

TURNER'S SYNDROME

Females with XO chromosome constitution, webbed neck, diminished growth, mental retardation, coarctation of aorta, hypertelorism, ptosis, epicanthal folds, and cataracts.

USHER'S SYNDROME

Retinitis pigmentosa, deafness, and mutism.

VOGT-KOYANAGI-HARADA SYNDROME

Primarily seen in more darkly pigmented individuals, poliosis, vitiligo, headache, tinnitus or other hearing defects, meningeal irritation, headache, seizure disorder, bilateral uveitis, serous retinal or choroidal detachments, exudative choroiditis, and cataracts.

VON HIPPEL-LINDAU SYNDROME

Retinal angiomas, cerebellar hemangiomas, visceral organ malformations, and pheochromocytomas.

WEBER'S SYNDROME

Third nerve palsy with contralateral hemiplegia and paralysis of face.

WEILL-MARCHESANI SYNDROME

Microsperophakia, subluxed lens, and short and stalky habitus.

WYBURN-MASON SYNDROME

Retinal arteriovenous communications, midbrain arteriovenous malformation, and intracranial calcification.

NOTES

20

Typical Laser Settings for Select Ophthalmic Procedures

The typical starting laser settings are listed below. Typically the power will need to be titrated upward from these settings until the desired effect is reached. The final proper laser settings are both laser and patient dependent.

FOCAL TREATMENT FOR MACULAR EDEMA

	Argon-Green	Yellow Dye
Spot size	50–100 μm	50 μm
Duration	0.1 sec	0.1 sec
Power	100 mW	70 mW

Increase power by 50 mW until there is visible whitening or color change of the lesion (microaneurysm). Do not treat hemorrhages. Treating with too much power or over the hemorrhage can lead to choroidal neovascularization. Treat all lesions 500–3,000 μm from the macular center that are thought to be causing macular edema.

If macular edema persists, vision is less than 20/40, and there is a good perifoveal capillary network, microaneurysms 300–500 μm from the macular center can be treated.

Large microaneurysms can be closed with several 50-μm burns. Small microaneurysms further than 500 μm from the macular center can be pretreated with a 100-μm spot to prevent subsequent burns from penetrating into the retinal pigment epithelium. Closure can then be accomplished with a 50-μm spot.

MACULAR GRID

	Argon-Green
Spot size	100–200 μm (50 μm in highly thickened retina)
Duration	≤0.1 sec
Power	100 mW

Increase power by 50 mW until there is a light retinal burn. As in focal treatment above, avoid hemorrhages and very white burns. Apply laser in a grid over thickened retina by spacing the burns one burn-width apart. Avoid treatment closer than 500 μm from the macular center or closer than 500 μm to the optic disc margin.

FOCAL TREATMENT OF A CHOROIDAL NEOVASCULAR MEMBRANE

Outline of Lesion

	Argon-Green
Spot size	100 μm
Duration	0.2 sec
Power	100 mW

Fill-In

	Argon-Green
Spot size	200–500 μm
Duration	0.5 sec
Power	100 mW

Perform outline of lesion just beyond the edge of the net as mapped with a fluorescein angiogram (unless the fovea is involved, in which case treatment is just to the edge of the net on the foveal side. Fill-in is accomplished with overlapping, confluent burns. The goal is bright whitening of the lesion and overlying retina. Increase the laser power as necessary until this is accomplished.

PANRETINAL PHOTOCOAGULATION

	Argon-Green
Spot size	200 μm (with Rodenstock or QuadrAspheric contact lens)
	500 μm (with Goldmann three-mirror lens)
Duration	0.1 sec
Power	100 mW

Increase power in approximately 50-mW steps until there is mild retinal whitening. The goal is approximately 2,000 spots spaced approximately one burn-width apart over three treatment sessions. Avoid treating within 4 DD temporal to the fovea and within the vascular arcades. Avoid treating within 1 DD of the optic disc. Avoid treating over major vessels or hemorrhage. Be diligent about knowing where the fovea is and avoid "losing your bearings." Retrobulbar or peribulbar anesthesia may be necessary for pain control. Subsequent fill-in treatment involves, as you would guess, treatment of retina between previous burn scars.

LASER SUTURE LYSIS

Spot size	100 μm
Duration	0.1 sec
Power	350–500 mW

Place the aiming beam over the laser after compressing the overlying conjunctiva with a Hoskins lens or the edge of a Zeiss 4 mirror contact lens.

LASER TRABECULOPLASTY

Spot size	50 μm
Duration	0.1 sec
Power	500–800 mW

Generally performed by placing 50 equally spaced burns over 180–360 degrees of the angle with a Goldmann three-mirror lens at the junction of the posterior pigmented and anterior nonpigmented trabecular meshwork. The goal is bubble formation or slight blanching. Pretreatment and post-treatment with apraclonidine is commonly performed in an attempt to prevent postoperative pressure spikes. Intraocular pressure is checked 1 hour after treatment. Low-dose steroids (e.g., fluorometholone 0.1% qid) can be prescribed for the first week after treatment to control inflammation and prevent peripheral synechiae.

YAG CAPSULOTOMY

Power	1–2 mJ
Shots per burst	1

Pretreatment and post-treatment with apraclonidine is common. Perform with or without Abraham lens. Aim on or just posterior to the posterior capsule. Check intraocular pressure 1 hour after procedure.

PERIPHERAL IRIDOTOMY: YAG LASER

Power	3–5 mJ
Shots per burst	1–3

Most effective with a contact lens to focus the laser. Pick a spot in the superior peripheral iris, where there is some room between the iris and cornea. Some clinicians choose to pretreat with an argon laser to prevent bleeding. If bleeding does result, place pressure on the globe by pressing with the contact lens. Aim just deep to the iris surface. Increase the power in 1- to 2-mJ increments until the iridotomy is patent. Penetration through the iris is usually recognized by a gush of aqueous and pigment from the iridotomy sight. Continued pulses through a patent iridotomy can result in zonular dehiscence and/or cataract formation.

YAG VITREOLYSIS

Power	3–6 mJ
Shots per burst	1

Pretreatment and post-treatment with apraclonidine or other glaucoma medication is common. Place aiming beam directly on vitreous strand.

NOTES

21

Commonly Used Ophthalmic Abbreviations

ABK	aphakic bullous keratopathy
AC	anterior chamber
AION	anterior ischemic optic neuropathy
ALT	argon laser trabeculoplasty
AMD	age-related macular degeneration
APD	afferent pupillary defect
ARMD	age-related macular degeneration
BDR	background diabetic retinopathy
BLR	bilateral recession or resection
BMR	bimedial recession or resection
BRAO	branch retinal artery occlusion
BRVO	branch retinal vein occlusion
BS	blind spot
C	cell
cc	with correction
C/D	cup-to-disc ratio
CF	count fingers
C/F	cell and flare
CL	contact lens
CME	cystoid macular edema
CMV	cytomegalovirus
CNVM	choroidal neovascular membrane
COAG	chronic open-angle glaucoma
CRAO	central retinal artery occlusion

CRVO	central retinal vein occlusion
CSME	clinically significant macular edema
DCR	dacryocystorhinostomy
ECCE	extracapsular cataract extraction
EKC	epidemic keratoconjunctivitis
EOM	extraocular muscles (or motility)
F	flare
FA	fluorescein angiography
FTFC	full to finger count
gtt	drop
GVF	Goldmann visual field
H:	Hertel exophthalmometry
HA	Henry Allen cards (or homatropine)
HM	hand motion
HVF	Humphrey visual fields
ICCE	Intracapsular cataract extraction
IK	interstitial keratitis
IOP	intraocular pressure
IRMA	intraretinal microvascular abnormality
JXG	juvenile xanthogranuloma
K	cornea
K:	keratometry
KP	keratic precipitate
K sicca	keratoconjunctivitis sicca
LF	levator function
LK	lamellar keratoplasty
LLL	lids, lashes, lacrimal (or left lower lid)
LP	light perception
LPI	laser peripheral iridotomy
LUL	left upper lid
M	macula
MRD	marginal reflex distance
MRx:	manifest refraction
NAG	narrow angle glaucoma
NLD	nasolacrimal duct

NLP	no light perception
NS	nuclear sclerosis
NVD	neovascularization of the disc
NVE	neovascularization elsewhere
OHS	ocular histoplasmosis syndrome
OHT	ocular hypertension
ON	optic nerve
ONH	optic nerve head
PAS	peripheral anterior synechiae
PBK	pseudophakic bullous keratopathy
PC	posterior capsule
PDR	proliferative diabetic retinopathy
PF	palpebral fissure
PG	patient's glasses
PH	pinhole
PHPV	persistent hyperplastic vitreous
PI	peripheral iridectomy (-otomy)
PK	penetrating keratoplasty
POAG	primary open angle glaucoma
POHS	presumed ocular histoplasmosis syndrome
PPDR	preproliferative diabetic retinopathy
PPV(tx)	pars plana vitrectomy
PRK	photorefractive keratectomy
PRP	panretinal photocoagulation
PS	posterior synechiae
PSC	posterior subcapsular cataract
PVD	posterior vitreous detachment
PVS	posterior vitreous separation
PVR	proliferative vitreoretinopathy
R:	retinoscopy
RLF	retrolental fibroplasia
ROP	retinopathy of prematurity
RP	retinitis pigmentosa
RPE	retinal pigmented epithelium
sc	without correction

SLE	slit lamp exam
SLK	superior limbic keratoconjunctivitis
SPK	superficial punctate keratitis
SRNV	subretinal neovascularization
Ta:	applanation tonometry
TM	trabecular meshwork
ung	ointment
V	vitreous or vessels
VA	visual acuity
VF	visual field
V(t)x	vitrectomy
W & Q	white and quiet

NOTES

22

Ophthalmic Pharmaceuticals

Table 22.1 Topical Antibacterial Agents

Generic Name Trade Name (Size)	Susceptible Organisms	Notes
Bacitracin (3.5 g)	Gram-positive, *Haemophilus influenzae, Treponema pallidum, Entamoeba histolytica, Actinomyces, Fusobacterium*	Available in ointment only.
Chloramphenicol Ak-Chlor (7.5–15.0 ml or 3.5 g) Chloroptic (7.5 ml or 3.5 g), Ocu-Chlor (7.5–15.0 ml or 3.5 g), Ophthochlor (15 ml)	Most gram-positive and gram-negative organisms, *H. influenzae, Staphylococcus aureus, Streptococcus hemolyticus, Neisseria* sp., *Escherichia coli, Klebsiella* and *Enterobacter* spp., and *Moraxella lacunata.* Not *Pseudomonas* or *Serratia marcescens*	Cases of bone marrow aplasia (1 fatal) have been reported following prolonged or frequent topical use.
Ciprofloxacin Ciloxan (2.5–5.0 ml, 3.5 g)	Wide range, fluoroquinolone active against *S. aureus, Staphylococcus epidermidis, Streptococcus viridans, Streptococcus pneumoniae,* and *Pseudomonas* and *Serratia* spp.	Indicated for the topical treatment of corneal ulcers by susceptible organisms. Associated with a reversible, superficial, white, crystalline infiltrate. Safety and efficacy in children under 12 not established.

Generic Name Trade Name (Size)	Susceptible Organisms	Notes
Erythromycin Ilotycin (3.5 g)	Wide range, especially against gram-positive organisms. Some strains of *H. influenza* and *S. aureus* are resistant. Used for prophylaxis of ophthalmia neonatorum due to *Neisseria* and *Chlamydia* spp.	Available in ointment only.
Gentamicin sulfate Genoptic (5 ml or 3.5 g) Gentak (5–15 ml or 3.5 g) Garamycin (5 ml or 3.5 g) Ocu-Mycin (5–15 ml or 3.5 g)	*Staphylococcus*, group A streptococci, diplococcus pneumoniae, strains of *Pseudomonas, Proteus, Klebsiella pneumoniae, H. influenzae* and *aegyptus, M. lacunata, E. coli,* and *Neisseria* sp. Some strains of *S. pneumoniae* are resistant.	Similar spectrum to tobramycin.
Neomycin/polymyxin B/ bacitracin-gramicidin Ocutricin (2–10 ml or 3.5 g) Neosporin (10 ml or 3.5 g) AK-Spore (2–10 ml or 3.5 g) Ocu-Spore (10 ml or 3.5 g)	These triple antibiotics use gramicidin in solution and bacitracin in ointment. Effective against most ocular pathogens, including: *S. aureus, Streptococcus, E. coli, H. influenzae, Klebsiella, Enterobacter, Neisseria,* and *Pseudomonas* spp. Not *S. marcescens.*	Associated with a 5–10% incidence of delayed hypersensitivity reactions to neomycin.
Norfloxacin Chibroxin (5 ml)	Synthetic broad-spectrum antibiotic (fluoroquinolone). Active against penicillinase-producing and methicillin-resistant *S. aureus, S. pneumon-*	Similar to ciprofloxacin.

Generic Name Trade Name (Size)	Susceptible Organisms	Notes
	iae, and *H. influenzae*. Not effective in infections by obligate anaerobes.	
Ofloxacin Ocuflox (5 ml)	Synthetic quinolone. Active against *S. aureus* and *S. epidermidis, S. pneumoniae, Haemophilus, Proteus,* and *Pseudomonas* spp. and *Enterobacter cloacae*.	Similar to other quinolones. See Norfloxacin above.
Polymyxin B/bacitracin Polysporin (all 3.5 g) Ocumycin, AK-Polybac	Gram-positives, including hemolytic streptococci; gram-negatives, including *Pseudomonas* sp. and *H. influenzae*.	Available in ointment only.
Sulfacetamide sodium Bleph-10 (5–15 ml or 3.5 g) AK-Sulf (10% and 30%) Cetamide 10% ointment Isopto cetamide 15% solution Sulamyd 10% and 30% (5–15 ml or 3.5 g) Vasosulf 15% (5–15 ml)	Effective against gram-positives and gram-negatives including pyogenic cocci, gonococcus, *E. coli*, Koch-Weeks bacillus. **Significant percentage of staphylococci are resistant.**	Allergic sensitization not uncommon. Not for use with very purulent infections.
Sulfisoxazole diolamine Gantrisin (15 ml or 3.5 g)	Similar properties to sulfacetamide (see above).	—
Tetracycline Achromycin (4 ml or 3.5 g) Aureomycin (3.5 g)	Susceptible organisms include *S. aureus, Streptococcus, E. coli, Neisseria* sp., *Chlamydia*. Useful in prophylaxis of ophthalmia neonatorum due to *Neisseria gonorrhoeae* and *Chlamydia*.	Oral agents necessary for adult inclusion conjunctivitis.
Tobramycin Tobrex (5 ml or 3.5 g)	Gram-positive and gram-negative organisms, including *Staphy-*	Similar to gentamicin but less likely to cause hypersensitivity.

Generic Name Trade Name (Size)	Susceptible Organisms	Notes
	lococcus, some *Strepto- coccus, E. coli, Kleb- siella* and *Enterobacter, Proteus, H. influenzae, H. aegyptus, M. lacu- nata*, some *Neisseria*. Less resistance com- pared to gentamicin.	
Trimethoprim sulfate/ polmyxin B Polytrim (10 ml)	Gram-positive and gram- negative organisms, including *Staphylo- coccus, Streptococcus, H. influenzae, H. aegyp- tus, S. marcescens, Pro- teus, Enterobacter, Klebsiella, E. coli*, and *Pseudomonas*.	Excellent spectrum of activity. Low rate of sensitivity (2%). Bac- teriostatic.

Table 22.2   Systemic Antimicrobial Agents

Generic Name Trade Name	Clinical Indications	Normal Dosage
Acyclovir Zovirax	Herpes zoster	800 mg PO 5 times a day for 7–10 days
	Herpes simplex	200 mg PO 5 times a day for 7–10 days
	ARN/PORN	10–20 mg/kg IV (adjusted for renal status) divided q8 for at least 7 days followed by PO 800 mg 5 times a day for 2–4 weeks
Amoxicillin	Endocarditis prophylaxis	3 g PO 1 hour before proce- dure, then 1.5 g PO 6 hours after procedure
Amoxicillin/Clavulanate Augmentin	Mild preseptal cellu- litis Dacryocystitis	250–500 mg PO q8h in adults or 20–40 mg/kg/day in 3 divided doses in chil- dren (over age 5)
Ampicillin	*Haemophilus* conjunc- tivitis in newborns	50–200 mg/kg IM or IV q12h for 10 days

Generic Name Trade Name	Clinical Indications	Normal Dosage
Ampicillin/ Sulbactam Unasyn	—	1.5–3.0 g IV q6h
Azithromycin Zithromax	Inclusion conjunctivitis *Chlamydia trachomatous*	20 mg/kg PO single dose*
Cefaclor Ceclor	Mild preseptal cellulitis	250–500 mg PO q8h in adults 20–40 mg/kg/day in 3 divided doses in children (over age 5)
Ceftazadime Fortaz	Preseptal cellulitis	30–50 mg/kg IV q8h in children (max. 6 g/day) or 1–2 g q8h in adults
Ceftriaxone Rocephin	Ophthalmia neona- torum due to gonococcus With nafcillin for orbital	125 mg IM in one dose 1 g IV q12–24h
Cephalexin Keflex	Dacryocystitis	500 mg PO q6h
Cidofovir Vistide	CMV retinitis	—
Ciprofloxacin Cipro	Cat scratch disease	500–750 mg PO q12h
Dicloxacillin	Dacryocystitis	500 mg PO q6h
Doxycycline	*Chlamydia* Lyme disease	100 mg PO bid for 3 weeks 100 mg PO bid for 10 days
Erythromycin	Ocular rosacea Inclusion conjunctivitis	250 mg PO qid
Famciclovir Famvir	Herpes zoster ophthalmicus	500 mg PO tid for 7 days
Fluconazole Diflucan	Canaliculitis from *Candida*	600 mg PO qd
Foscarnet Foscavir	Cytomegalovirus retinitis	Induction with 90 mg/kg (over 2 hrs) IV q12h for 14 days. Maintenance dose is 90–120 mg/kg once daily over 2 hrs
Ganciclovir Cytovene	Cytomegalovirus retinitis	5 mg/kg IV over 1 hr q12h for 14–21 days (induction). Maintenance dose is 5 mg/kg once daily over 1 hr q24h or 1,000 mg PO tid with food (250-mg tablets)

Generic Name Trade Name	Clinical Indications	Normal Dosage
Nafcillin	Along with ceftriaxone for orbital cellulitis	1–2g IV q4h
Oxacillin	Preseptal cellulitis	150 mg/kg/day IV in 6 divided doses in children, or 1–2 g q4h in adults
Penicillin V	Canaliculitis from *Actinomyces*	500 mg PO qid
Tetracycline	Ocular rosacea Inclusion conjunctivitis	250 mg PO qid
Trimethoprim/ sulfamethoxazole Bactrim	Mild preseptal cellulitis	160/800 mg PO bid in adults 8/40 mg/kg/day in 2 divided doses in children (over age 5)
Valacyclovir Valtrex	Herpes zoster	1g PO tid for 7 days

*Not an FDA-approved indication.

Table 22.3   Topical Antibacterial Agents with Steroids

Trade Name	Antibacterial Agents	Steroids
Blephamide (2.5–10.0 ml)	Sulfacetamide	Prednisolone acetate 0.2%
Blephamide ointment (3.5 g)	Sulfacetamide	Prednisolone acetate 0.2%
Chloromycetin (5 ml)	Chloramphenicol	Hydrocortisone 2.5%
Cortisporin (7.5 ml)	Polymyxin B, neomycin	Hydrocortisone 1%
Cortisporin ointment (3.5g)	Polymyxin B, neomycin, bacitracin	Hydrocortisone 1%
Dexacidin (5 ml)	Polymyxin B, neomycin	Dexamethasone 0.1%
Dexacidin ointment (3.5 g)	Polymyxin B, neomycin	Dexamethasone 0.1%
FML-S	Sulfacetamide	Fluormetholone
Maxitrol (5 ml)	Polymyxin B, neomycin	Dexamethasone 0.1%
Maxitrol ointment (3.5 g)	Polymyxin B, neomycin	Dexamethasone 0.1%
Metimyd (5 ml)	Sulfacetamide	Prednisolone acetate 0.5%

Trade Name	Antibacterial Agents	Steroids
Metimyd ointment (3.5 g)	Sulfacetamide	Prednisolone acetate 0.5%
NeoDecadron (5 ml)	Neomycin	Dexamethasone 0.1%
NeoDecadron ointment (3.5 g)	Neomycin	Dexamethasone 0.1%
Ophthocort (3.5 g)	Chloramphenicol, polymyxin B	Hydrocortisone 0.5%
Polypred (5 ml)	Polymyxin B, neomycin	Prednisolone acetate 0.5%
Pred-G (5–10 ml)	Gentamicin	Prednisolone acetate 1.0%
Tobradex (5 ml)	Tobramycin	Dexamethasone 0.1%
Tobradex ointment (3.5 g)	Tobramycin	Dexamethasone 0.1%
Vasocidin (5–10 ml)	Sulfacetamide	Prednisolone phosphate 0.25%
Vasocidin ointment (3.5 g)	Sulfacetamide	Prednisolone acetate 0.5%

Table 22.4   Topical Corticosteroids

Generic Name	Concentration (%)	Trade Name
Dexamethasone phosphate solution	0.1	Ak-Dex (5 ml); Decadron (5 ml)
Dexamethasone phosphate ointment	0.05	Ak-Dex (3.5 g); Decadron (3.5 g)
Dexamethasone alcohol solution	0.1	Maxidex (5–15 ml)
Dexamethasone alcohol ointment	0.05	Maxidex (3.5 g)
Fluorometholone suspension	0.1	FML (5–15 ml)
Fluorometholone suspension	0.25	FML Forte (5 ml)
Fluorometholone ointment	0.1	FML (3.5 g)
Fluorometholone acetate	0.1	Flarex
Loteprednol etabonate	0.5	Lotemax (2.5, 5, 10, 15 ml)
	0.2	Alrex (5, 10 ml)
Medrysone	1.0	HMS (5–10 ml)
Prednisolone acetate suspension	0.125	Pred mild, Econopred (5–10 ml)
	1.0	Pred forte, Econopred plus (5–10 ml)
Prednisolone sodium phosphate solution	0.125	Inflamase mild (5–10 ml); AK-Pred 0.125%
	1.0	Inflamase (5–10 ml); AK-Pred 1% (5–15 ml)
Rimexalone	1.0	Vexol

Table 22.5   Topical Antiviral Agents

Generic Name	Trade Names	Normal Dosage for Epithelial Disease
Idoxuridine	Herplex (15 ml) Stoxil (15 ml)	1 drop every hour (every 2 hrs at night)
	Stoxil ointment (4 g)	Instill 5 times a day
Vidarabine	Vira-A ointment (3.5 g)	Apply one-half inch 5 times a day
Trifluridine	Viroptic (7.5 ml)	1 drop every 2 hrs (max. of 9 times a day)

Table 22.6   Topical Antifungal Agents

Generic Name	Trade Name	Indications and Normal Dosage
Natamycin	Natacyn	Fungal blepharitis, conjunctivitis, and keratitis caused by susceptible organisms 1 drop 4–6 times a day for blepharitis/ conjunctivitis Hourly instillation for fungal keratitis

Table 22.7   Topical Nonsteroidal Anti-Inflammatory Drugs

Trade Name	Generic Name	Indications and Notes
Acular/Acular PF (preservative free)	Ketorolac tromethamine 0.5%	For relief of ocular itching due to seasonal allergic conjunctivitis. Contraindicated in patients while wearing soft contact lenses. One drop 4 times a day.
Ocufen*	Flurbiprofen 0.03%	Inhibition of intraoperative miosis. One drop q30min starting 2 hrs before surgery.
Profenal*	Suprofen 1%	Inhibition of intraoperative miosis. Two drops qh starting 3 hrs before surgery. May also apply 2 drops q4h while awake the day before surgery.
Voltaren	Diclofenac sodium 0.1%	Treatment of postoperative inflam- mation after cataract surgery (qid for 2 wks after surgery).

*Ocufen and Profenal are contraindicated in herpes simplex keratitis.

Table 22.8   Glaucoma Medications

CATEGORY *Generic Name* *Trade Name* *(Size)*	*Normal Dosage*	*Contraindications (C)* *and Side Effects (S)*
BETA BLOCKERS **Betaxolol** Betoptic (2.5, 5.0, and 10.0 ml) Betoptic-S (suspension) (2.5, 5.0, and 10.0 ml)	1 drop twice a day	C: sinus bradycardia, greater than first-degree atrioventricular block, cardiogenic shock, overt cardiac failure S: stinging on instillation, itching, keratitis; rarely insomnia, breathing difficulties in patients with preexisting restriction of pulmonary function
Carteolol Ocupress 1%	1 drop twice daily	C: same as betaxolol plus: asthma or chronic obstructive pulmonary disease S: ocular irritation, blurry vision, photophobia, decreased night vision, blepharoconjunctivitis, ptosis, arrythmias, hypotension, dyspnea, dizziness, headache, insomnia
Levobunolol Betagan 0.25% and 0.5% (5–10 ml)	1 drop 1–2 times a day	C: same as betaxolol plus asthma or chronic obstructive pulmonary disease S: burning and stinging, decreased heart rate and blood pressure, headache, arrhythmia, bronchospasm, respiratory failure, depression
Metipranolol Optipranolol 0.3% (2, 5, and 10 ml)	1 drop twice a day	C: same as levobunolol S: same as levobunolol plus granulomatous iritis

CATEGORY *Generic Name* Trade Name *(Size)*	*Normal Dosage*	*Contraindications (C)* *and Side Effects (S)*
Timolol		C: same as levobunolol
Timoptic 0.25% and 0.5%	1 drop twice a day	S: same as levobunolol
Betimol 0.5% (5, 10, and 15 ml)	1 drop twice a day	Note that 1 in 3 patients has transient visual blurring lasting 30 secs to 5 mins immediately after instilla-
Timoptic-XE 0.25% and 0.5%	1 drop once a day	tion with Timoptic-XE
MIOTICS		
Pilocarpine		C: acute iritis
Various trade names 1%, 2%, 4%, and 6%* (15 ml)	1 drop 1–4 times a day	S: ciliary spasm, headache, lacrimation, induced
Ocusert Pilo (20 and 40)	1 unit per week	myopia, reduced acuity; may induce retinal
Pilopine HS gel (5 g)	½-in. ribbon at bedtime	detachment, lens opaci- ties with prolonged use; systemic complications are rare
Pilocarpine with epinephrine (see Epinephrine under Adrenergic Agonists)		
Pilocarpine and physostigmine		Studies indicate no addi- tive therapeutic effect
Isopto P-ES (15 ml)	1–2 drops up to 4 times a day	over either agent used alone; combination not recommended
Carbachol		C: same as pilocarpine
Isoptocarbachol 0.75%, 1.5%, 2.25%, and 3.0% (15 ml)	1–2 drops up to 3 times a day	S: same as pilocarpine plus salivation, syncope, car- diac arrhythmia, cramping, vomiting, asthma, diarrhea
Isoflurophate		C: iritis, angle closure,
Floropryl ointment (3.5 g)	¼-in. ribbon every third day up to 3 times a day	pregnancy; use with cau- tion in patients with con- ditions that may respond to vagotonic effect
Demecarium bromide		This is an extremely
Humorsol 0.125% and 0.25%	1–2 drops twice a week to twice a day	potent drug; please read PDR or package insert before initiating therapy

CATEGORY Generic Name Trade Name (Size)	Normal Dosage	Contraindications (C) and Side Effects (S)
Physostigmine Eserine 0.25% (3.5 g)	Apply 1–3 times a day	C: same as isoflurophate S: same as isoflurophate
Ecothiophate iodide Phospholine iodide 0.03%, 0.06%, 0.125%, and 0.25% (5 ml)	1 drop 1–2 times a day	C: same as isoflurophate S: same as isoflurophate
ADRENERGIC AGONISTS		
Apraclonidine Iopidine 1% (0.25 ml)	1 drop 1 hr prior and immediately after laser surgery	For prevention of post-laser pressure spikes C: hypersensitivity to this medication or to clonidine S: mydriasis, lid retraction, bradycardia, vasovagal reaction, palpitations, orthostatic hypotension, insomnia, decreased libido, gastrointestinal reactions
Iopidine 0.5% (5 ml)	1 drop 2–3 times a day	Same contraindications and side effects as 1% formulation. Local allergic reactions not uncommon.
Brimonidine Alphagan	1 drop twice a day	C: patients with sensitivity to brimonidine. Patients on monoamine oxidase therapy. S: dry mouth, ocular hyperemia, burning and stinging, foreign body sensation. Ocular allergic reactions.
Epinephrine Epifrin 0.25%, 0.5%, 1%, and 2% (15 ml) Glaucon 1% and 2% (10 ml)	1 drop 1–2 times a day	C: narrow-angle, hypersensitivity to any ingredient, aphakia; use with caution in hyperthyroidism, hypertension, cardiac

CATEGORY **Generic Name** **Trade Name** (bottle or tube size)	*Normal Dosage*	*Contraindications (C)* *and Side Effects (S)*
Eppy/N 0.5%, 1%, and 2% (7.5 ml)		disease, long-standing bronchial asthma S: hypertension, tachycardia, angina, nosebleeds, staining of soft contact lenses, conjunctival pigmentation
Epinephrine and pilocarpine E-Pilo-1, -2, -3, -4, -6 (10 ml) P1E1, P2E1, P3E1, P4E1, P6E1 (15 ml)	1 drop 2 times a day 1 drop 2 times a day	C: this is a combination of epinephrine and pilocarpine; contraindications and side effects of both apply
Dipivefrin Propine 0.1% (5, 10, and 15 ml)	1 drop 2 times a day	C: same as epinephrine S: same as epinephrine but less likely or less severe
PROSTAGLANDIN ANALOGS **Latanoprost 0.005%** Xalatan (2.5 ml)	1 drop qhs	C: sensitivity to active ingredient. S: burning and stinging, conjunctival hyperemia, itching, punctate keratopathy, skin rash. Iris color changes may be permanent. Increased length, thickness of lashes. Recurrent cystoid macular edema.
TOPICAL CARBONIC ANHYDRASE INHIBITORS **Brinzolamide 1%** Azopt (10 ml)	1 drop 3 times daily	C: allergy to brinzolamide S: burning, itching, dry mouth
Dorzolamide 2% Trusopt (10 ml)	1 drop 3 times daily	C: allergy S: punctate keratitis, lethargy, GI upset,

CATEGORY Generic Name Trade Name (bottle or tube size)	Normal Dosage	Contraindications (C) and Side Effects (S)
		Stevens-Johnson (this is a sulfa compound); same side effects as oral carbonic anhydrase inhibitors except less common and less severe.
Dorzolamide/timolol Cosopt	1 drop 2 times a day	Same contraindications and side effects as each drug individually.
SYSTEMIC CARBONIC ANHYDRASE INHIBITORS **Acetazolamide** Diamox 125-, 250-mg tablets 500-mg sequels IV/IM	2–4 times a day 1–2 times a day 500 mg (can repeat in 2–4 hrs)	C: depressed sodium/potassium serum levels, marked kidney and liver disease, hyperchloremic acidosis; use lower doses in renal impairment S: paresthesias, tingling in extremities, appetite loss, polyuria, lethargy, potentiates renal stone formation. Rarely hemolytic anemia, bone marrow depression, thrombocytopenic purpura, Stevens-Johnson syndrome
Methazolamide Neptazane MZM (25-, 50-mg tablets)	50–200 mg a day in 2–3 divided doses	C: same as acetazolamide except the incidence of renal stone formation may be less S: same as acetazolamide; some patients who cannot tolerate Diamox may be able to tolerate Neptazane

CATEGORY *Generic Name* *Trade Name* *(bottle or tube size)*	*Normal Dosage*	*Contraindications (C)* *and Side Effects (S)*
Dichlorphenamide Daranide (50-mg tablets)	1–2 tablets, 1–2 times a day	C: same as acetazolamide S: same as acetazolamide
SYSTEMIC OSMOTIC AGENTS **Glycerine** Osmoglyn 50%	2–3 ml/kg PO (approx. 4–6 oz)	C: well-established anuria, severe dehydration, frank or impending acute pulmonary edema, severe cardiac decompensation. Use with caution in diabetics. S: nausea, vomiting, headache, confusion, disorientation; severe dehydration, cardiac arrhythmia, hyperosmolar nonketotic coma that can result in death
Isosorbide 45% Ismotic (220 ml)	1.5 g/kg PO	Similar to Osmoglyn (above) but does not affect blood glucose; less nausea and vomiting; more significant diuresis.
Mannitol Osmitrol	0.5–2.0 g/kg IV infused over 30–60 mins q6–8h	C: congestive heart failure. S: headache, nausea, vomiting, dehydration, massive diuresis, chills, dizziness, chest pain, agitation, disorientation, convulsions. Can cause pulmonary edema and intracranial hemorrhage.

*Other concentrations available but rarely used.

Table 22.9   Artificial Tears

Trade Name	Major Component	Preservatives
Adsorbotear	Hydroxyethylcellulose/povidone	Thimerasol/edetate disodium
Bion Tears	Dextran 70%, Hydroxypropyl methylcellulose	—
Cellufresh	Carboxymethylcellulose 0.5%	—
Celluvisc	Carboxymethylcellulose 1%	—
Comfort Tears	Hydroxyethylcellulose	BAK/edetate disodium
Dry Eye Therapy	Glycerin 0.3%	—
GenTeal	Hydroxypropyl methylcellulose	Sodium perborate
Hypotears	Polyvinyl alcohol	BAK/edetate disodium
Hypotears PF	Polyvinyl alcohol and lipiden	—
Isopto Tears	Hydroxypropyl methylcellulose	BAK
Just Tears	Hydroxypropyl methylcellulose	BAK/edetate disodium
Lacril	Hydroxypropyl methylcellulose	Chlorobutanol
Lacrisert (inserts)	Hydroxypropyl cellulose	—
Liquifilm Forte	Polyvinyl alcohol	Thimerasol/edetate disodium
Liquifilm Tears	Polyvinyl alcohol	Chlorobutanol
Moisture Drops	Hydroxypropyl methylcellulose Dextran 40	BAK/edetate disodium
Moisture Eyes	Propylene glycol	—
Murine	Polyvinyl alcohol/povidone	BAK/edetate disodium
Murocel	Methylcellulose	Methylparaben/ propylparaben
Neo-Tears	Polyvinyl alcohol/cellulose ester	Thimerasol/edetate disodium
Refresh	Polyvinyl alcohol/povidone	—
Refresh Plus	Carboxymethylcellulose 0.5%	—
Refresh Tears	Carboxymethylcellulose 0.5%	Purite
TearGard	Hydroxyethylcellulose	Sorbic acid/edetate disodium
Tearisol	Hydroxypropyl methylcellulose	BAK/edetate disodium
Tears Naturale II	Hydroxypropyl methylcellulose	Polyquad/edetate disodium
Tears Naturale Free	Hydroxypropylmethylcellulose/ dextran	—
Tears Plus	Polyvinyl alcohol/povidone	Chlorobutanol
Tears Renewed	Hydroxypropyl methylcellulose	BAK/edetate disodium
Vit-A-Drops	Vitamin A, polysorbate 80	Ethylenediamine- tetraacetic acid

Table 22.10   Bland Ophthalmic Ointments

Trade Name	Major Component	Preservatives
Akwa-Tears	Petrolatum/mineral oil/lanolin	—
Dry Eyes	Petrolatum/mineral oil/lanolin	—
Duolube	Petrolatum/mineral oil	—
Duratears	Petrolatum/mineral oil/lanolin	Methylparaben/ polyparaben
Hypotears	Petrolatum/mineral oil	—
Lacri-Lube	Petrolatum/mineral oil/lanolin	Chlorobutanol
Lacri-Lube NP	Petrolatum/mineral oil/lanolin	—
LubriTears	Petrolatum/mineral oil/lanolin	Chlorobutanol
Oculube	Petrolatum/mineral oil	—
Refresh PM	Petrolatum/mineral oil	—

Table 22.11   Topical Hyperosmotic Agents

Trade Name	Sodium Chloride Concentration	Normal Dosage
Adsorbonac (15 ml)	2% and 5%	1–2 drops every 3–4 hrs
AK-NaCl (15 ml)	5%	1 or more times a day
AK-NaCl ointment (3.5 g)	5%	1 or more times a day
Muro-128 (15 ml)	2% and 5%	1–2 drops every 3–4 hrs
Muro-128 ointment (3.5 g)	5%	1 or more times a day
Ophthalgan	Glycerin	1–2 drops to clear edematous cornea prior to examination

Table 22.12   Topical Decongestants

Generic Name	Trade Name	Preservative
Naphazoline hydrochloride	Ak-Con	BAK and edetate disodium
	Albalon	BAK and edetate disodium
	Allerest	BAK and edetate disodium
	Clear Eyes	BAK and edetate disodium
	Comfort Eye Drops	BAK and edetate disodium
	Degest 2	BAK and edetate disodium
	Maximum Strength Allergy Drops	BAK and edetate disodium
	Muro's Opcon	BAK and edetate disodium
	Nafazair	BAK and edetate disodium
	Naphcon	BAK and edetate disodium
	Naphcon Forte	BAK and edetate disodium

Generic Name	Trade Name	Preservative
	Vasoclear	BAK and edetate disodium
	Vasocon Regular	BAK and edetate disodium
Oxymetazoline hydrochloride	OcuClear	BAK and edetate disodium
	Visine L.R.	BAK and edetate disodium
Phenylephrine hydrochloride	Ak-Nefrin	BAK and edetate disodium
	Isopto Frin	BAK
	Prefrin Liquifilm	BAK and edetate disodium
	Relief	Preservative free
Tetrahydrozoline hydrochloride	Collyrium	BAK and edetate disodium
	Murine Plus	BAK and edetate disodium
	Soothe	BAK and edetate disodium
	Tetrasine	BAK and edetate disodium
	Visine	BAK and edetate disodium
	Visine Extra	BAK and edetate disodium

Table 22.13   Decongestants and Astringents

Generic Name	Trade Name	Preservative
Phenylephrine hydrochloride and zinc sulfate	Prefrin-Z	Thimerosal
	Zincfrin	BAK and polysorbate 80
Tetrahydrozaline and zinc sulphate	Visine A.C.	BAK and edetate disodium

Table 22.14   Antihistamines and Decongestants

Trade Name	Decongestant	Antihistamine	Preservative
Ak-Con-A	Naphazoline hydrochloride	Pheniramine maleate	BAK
Albalon-A	Naphazoline hydrochloride	Antazoline phosphate	BAK
Emadine	—	Emedastine difumarate	—
Livostin	—	Levocobastine	—
Muro's Opcon-A	Naphazoline hydrochloride	Pheniramine maleate	BAK
Nafazair	Naphazoline hydrochloride	Pheniramine maleate	—
Naphcon-A	Naphazoline hydrochloride	Pheniramine maleate	BAK

Trade Name	Decongestant	Antihistamine	Preservative
Patanol* (5 ml)	—	Olopatadine hydrochloride	—
Phenylephrine	Pyrilamine hydrochloride	Pyrilamine maleate	BAK
Vasocon-A	Naphazoline hydrochloride	Antazoline phosphate	BAK

*Dual mechanism of action, antihistamine and mast cell stabilizer; usual dosage is 1–2 drops bid.

Table 22.15   Mydriatic and Cycloplegic Agents

Agent	Concentration
Mydriatic agents	
Phenylephrine	2.5% and 10%
Hydroxyamphetamine (Paredrine)	1%
Cycloplegic agents	
Atropine	0.5% and 1%
Homatropine	2% and 5%
Scopolamine	0.25%
Cyclopentolate	0.5%, 1%, and 2%
Tropicamide	0.5% and 1%

Table 22.16   Other Products

Trade Name	Generic Name	Description
Alomide	Lodoxamide tromethamine	Antiallergic mast cell stabilizer
Biocor 12, 24, and 72 Shields	Collagen corneal shields	Dissolvable contact lenses for trauma or surgery
Chiron Shields (24 h)	Collagen corneal shields	Same as above
Enuclene	Tyloxapol	Cleaning/lubricating agent for artificial eyes
EYE Scrub Cleanser	Disodium laureth	Cleansing pads for blepharitis, etc
EV Lid Cleanser	—	Similar to EYE Scrub above
Optichrome 4%	Cromolyn sodium	Antiallergic mast cell stabilizer
Rēv-Eyes	Dapiprazole hydrochloride	Used for reversal of mydriasis

Table 22.17 Selected Analgesic Agents

Trade Name *Schedule* *(if controlled)*	*Composition*	*Normal Dosage*
Acetaminophen	Acetaminophen 325-, 500-, or 650-mg tablets	500–1,000 mg PO q4–6h; max. is 4 g/day
	Chewable 80-mg tablet	2–3 yrs: 2 tablets; 4–5 yrs: 3 tablets; 6–8 yrs: 4 tablets; 9–10 yrs: 5 tablets; 11–12 yrs: 6 tablets q4h; max. of 5 doses/day
	Infant's suspension drops, 100 mg/ml	0–3 mos: 0.4 ml; 4–11 mos: 0.8 ml; 12–23 mos: 1.2 ml; 2–3 yrs: 1.6 ml; 4–5 yrs: 2.4 ml; q4h, max. 5 doses/day
	Children's elixir, 160 mg/5 ml	4–11 mos: 0.5 tsp.; 12–23 mos: 0.75 tsp.; 2–3 yrs: 1 tsp.; 4–5 yrs: 1.5 tsp.; 6–8 yrs: 2 tsp.; 9–10 yrs: 2.5 tsp.; 11–12 yrs: 3 tsp.; q4h, max. 5 doses/day
Advil	Ibuprofen 200-mg tablet	200 mg PO q4–6h
Codeine phospate C-II	Codeine phosphate	15–60 mg q4–6h IM, SC, or IV
Codeine sulfate C-II	Codeine sulfate 15-, 30-, and 60-mg tablets	15–60 mg PO q4–6h prn for pain
Darvocet-N 50 C-IV	Propoxyphene napsylate (50 mg) and acetaminophen (325 mg)	1–2 tablets PO q4h prn for pain
Darvocet-N 100 C-IV	Propoxyphene napsylate (100 mg) and acetaminophen (650 mg)	1 tablet PO q4h prn for pain
Darvon C-IV	Propoxyphene hydrochloride (65 mg)	1 tablet PO q4h prn for pain
Darvon-N C-IV	Propoxyphene napsylate 50 mg/5 ml suspension or 100-mg tablet	100 mg q4h prn for pain
Darvon compound-65 C-IV	Propoxyphene hydrochloride (65 mg), aspirin (389 mg), and caffeine (32.4 mg)	1 capsule PO q4h prn for pain
Demerol C-II	Meperidine hydrochloride 50- and 100-mg tablets	50–150 mg PO, IM, or SC q3–4h

Trade Name Schedule (if controlled)	Composition	Normal Dosage
Dilaudid C-II	Hydromorphone hydrochloride 1-, 2-, 3-, 4-mg tablets, parenteral	2 mg q4–6h PO prn for pain; 1–2 mg q4–6h SC or IM prn for pain
Fioricet	Acetaminophen (325 mg), butalbital (50 mg), and caffeine (40 mg)	1–2 tablets PO q4h prn, max. of 6 tablets a day
Fioricet with codeine C-III	Acetaminophen (325 mg), butalbital (50 mg), caffeine (40 mg), and codeine phosphate (30 mg)	1–2 tablets PO q4h prn, max. of 6 tablets a day
Fiorinal C-III	Aspirin (325 mg), butalbital (50 mg), and caffeine (40 mg)	1–2 tablets PO q4h prn, max. of 6 tablets a day
Fiorinal with codeine C-III	Aspirin (325 mg), butalbital (50 mg), caffeine (40 mg), and codeine phosphate (30 mg)	1–2 tablets PO q4h prn, max. of 6 tablets a day
Lodine	Etodolac 200-, 300-mg capsules	200–400 mg PO q6–8h
Lortab C-III	Per 5 ml: hydrocodone bitartrate (2.5 mg), acetaminophen (120 mg), and alcohol (7%)	15 ml PO q4h prn for pain
Lortab 2.5/500 C-III	Hydrocodone bitartrate (2.5 mg) and acetaminophen (500 mg)	1–2 tablets PO q4–6h prn for pain
Lortab 5/500 C-III	Hydrocodone bitartrate (5 mg) and acetaminophen (500 mg)	1–2 tablets PO q4–6h prn for pain
Lortab 7.5/500 C-III	Hydrocodone bitartrate (7.5 mg) and acetaminophen (500 mg)	1 tablet PO q4–6h prn for pain
Lortab ASA C-III	Hydrocodone bitartrate (5 mg) and aspirin (500 mg)	1–2 tablets PO q4–6h prn for pain
MS Contin C-II	Morphine sulfate 15-, 30-, 60-, 100-mg tablets	Variable
Motrin	Ibuprofen 300-, 400-, 600-, 800-mg tablets	400 mg PO q4–6h prn for pain
Naprosyn	Naproxen 250-, 375-, 500-mg tablets or 125 mg/5 ml suspension	500 mg PO then 250 mg q6–8h prn
Orudis	Ketoprofen 25-, 50-, 75-mg capsules	25–50 mg PO q6–8h
Pedioprofen	Ibuprofen 100 mg/5 ml	400 mg PO q4–6h prn for pain
Percocet C-II	Oxycodone hydrochloride (5 mg) and acetaminophen (325 mg)	1 tablet PO q6h prn for pain

Trade Name Schedule (if controlled)	Composition	Normal Dosage
Percodan C-II	Oxycodone hydrochloride (4.5 mg), oxycodone, terephthalate (0.19 mg), and aspirin (325 mg)	1 tablet PO q6h prn for pain
Stadol	Butorphanol tartrate injection	1 mg IV, 2 mg IM q3–4h prn for pain
	Nasal spray (10 mg/ml)	1 spray each nostril q3–4h prn
Talwin C-IV	Pentazocine (12.5 mg) and aspirin (325 mg)	1–2 caplets PO 3–4 times a day
Toradol	Ketorolac tromethamine 10-mg tablet and parenteral	1 tablet PO q6h prn for pain, or 30–60 mg IM loading, then half the loading dose q6h prn for pain
Tylenol	Acetaminophen 325-, 500-, or 650-mg tablets	500–1,000 mg PO q4–6h; max. 4 g/day. See Acetaminophen for children's dosages
Tylenol with codeine	Acetaminophen (300 mg) and	
#1 C-III	codeine phosphate (7.5 mg)	2–4 tablets PO q4h prn for pain
#2 C-III	codeine phosphate (15 mg)	2–3 tablets PO q4h prn for pain
#3 C-III	codeine phosphate (30 mg)	1–2 tablets PO q4h prn for pain
#4 C-III	codeine phosphate (60 mg)	1 tablet PO q4h prn for pain
Tylox C-II	Oxycodone (5 mg) and acetaminophen (500 mg)	1 caplet PO q6h prn for pain
Vicodin C-III	Hydrocodone bitartrate (5 mg) and acetaminophen (500 mg)	1–2 tablets PO q6h prn for pain
Vicodin ES C-III	Hydrocodone bitartrate (7.5 mg) and acetaminophen (750 mg)	1 tablet PO q4–6h prn for pain

Schedule I: No accepted medical abuse with high abuse potential.

Schedule II: High abuse potential. Possibility of severe psychological or physical dependence. Prescriptions must be written and personally signed. Not refillable.

Schedule III: Less abuse potential than schedule II. Low to moderate physical dependence. High psychological dependence. Prescriptions may be oral or written and are refillable up to five times in 6 months if authorized by the prescribing practitioner.

Schedule IV: Less abuse potential than schedule III. Limited physical or psychological dependence. Prescriptions may be oral or written and are refillable up to five times in 6 months if authorized by the prescribing practitioner.

Table 22.18   Prescription Abbreviations

bid	twice daily
caps	capsule
d	day
gt(t)	drop(s)
h	hr
hs	at bedtime
IM	intramuscular
IV	intravenous
PO	by mouth
prn	as needed
q	every
qid	4 times daily
SC	subcutaneous
tab	tablet
tid	3 times daily

Table 22.19   Color Codes for Topical Ocular Medications

Tan	Anti-infectives
Pink	Anti-inflammatories
Red	Mydriatic and cycloplegic agents
Gray	Nonsteroidal anti-inflammatory agents
Green	Miotic agents
Yellow or blue	Beta blockers
Purple	Adrenergic agonist agents
Orange	Carbonic anhydrase inhibitors
Turquoise	Prostaglandin analogues

Bibliography

American Academy of Ophthalmology. Basic and Clinical Science Course. Sections 1–12, 1996–97. San Francisco: American Academy of Ophthalmology, 1997.

Arffa RC. Grayson's Diseases of the Cornea (3rd ed). St. Louis: Mosby, 1991.

Bajandas FJ. Neuro-Ophthalmology Board Review Manual. Thorofare, NJ: Slack, 1980.

Beck RW. The optic neuritis treatment trial: implications for clinical practice. Arch Ophthalmol 1992;110:331–332.

Burde RM, Savino PJ, Trobe JD. Clinical Decisions in Neuro-Ophthalmology. St. Louis: Mosby, 1985.

Collins JF. Handbook of Clinical Ophthalmology. New York: Masson, 1982.

D'Amico DJ. Diseases of the retina. N Engl J Med 1994;331:95–106.

de la Maza MS, Jabbur NS, Foster CS. An analysis of therapeutic decision for scleritis. Ophthalmology 1993;100:1372–1376.

Derick RJ, Robin AL, Tielsch J et al. Once-daily versus twice-daily levobunolol (0.5%) therapy: a crossover study. Ophthalmology 1992;99:424–429.

DiGregorio GJ, Barbieri EJ. Handbook of Commonly Prescribed Drugs. (8th ed). West Chester, PA: Medical Surveillance, 1993.

Dornic DI. Acanthamoeba. In BE Onofrey (ed), Clinical Optometric Pharmacology and Therapeutics. Philadelphia: Lippincott, 1991.

Endophthalmitis Vitrectomy Study Group. Results of the Endophthalmitis Vitrectomy Study: a randomized trial of immediate vitrectomy and of intravenous antibiotics for the treatment of postoperative bacterial endophthalmitis. Arch Ophthalmol 1995;113:1479–1496.

Epstein DL. Chandler and Grant's Glaucoma (3rd ed). Philadelphia: Lea & Febiger, 1986.

Fraunfelder FT, Meyer SM. Drug-Induced Ocular Side Effects and Drug Interactions (2nd ed). Philadelphia: Lea & Febiger, 1982.

Fraunfelder FT, Roy FH. Current Ocular Therapy (3rd ed). Philadelphia: Saunders, 1990.

Friedberg MA, Rapuono CJ. Will's Eye Hospital Office and Emergency Room Diagnosis and Treatment of Eye Disease. Philadelphia: Lippincott, 1990.

Greenberg MS. Handbook of Neurosurgery (3rd ed). Lakeland, FL: Greenberg Graphics, 1994.

Gutman FA. Evaluation of a patient with central retinal vein occlusion. Ophthalmology 1983;90:481–483.

Hayreh SS. Classification of central retinal vein occlusion. Ophthalmology 1983;90:458–474.

Hobden JA, Reidy JJ, O'Callaghan RJ et al. Treatment of experimental pseudomonas keratitis using collagen shields containing tobramycin. Arch Ophthalmol 1988;106:1605–1607.

Hoskins HD, Kass M. Becker-Shaffer's Diagnosis and Therapy of the Glaucomas (6th ed). St. Louis: Mosby, 1989.

Kana JS. Delayed trifluridine treatment of subepithelial corneal infiltrates. Am J Ophthalmol 1992;113:212–214.

Kutner B, Fourman S, Brein K et al. Aminocaproic acid reduces the risk of secondary hemorrhage in patients with traumatic hyphema. Arch Ophthalmol 1987;105:206–208.

Martinez J, Smiddy WE, Kim J et al. Differentiating macular holes from macular pseudoholes. Am J Ophthalmol 1994;117:762–767.

Melles RB, Wong IG. Metipranol-associated granulomatous iritis. Am J Ophthalmol 1994;118:712–715.

Newell FW. Ophthalmology Principles and Concepts (7th ed). St. Louis: Mosby-Year Book, 1992.

Nozik RA, Schlaegel TF. Diagnostic Approach and Miscellaneous Analyses. In TD Duane (ed), Clinical Ophthalmology. Vol. 4. Philadelphia: Harper & Row, 1984.

O'Conner GR. Tests in Uveitis. In TD Duane (ed), Clinical Ophthalmology. Vol. 4. Philadelphia: Harper & Row, 1984.

O'Day DM, Jones BR. Herpes Simplex Keratitis. In TD Duane (ed), Clinical Ophthalmology. Vol. 4. Philadelphia: Harper & Row, 1984.

Olin BR. Drug Facts and Comparisons, 1995 Edition. St. Louis: Facts and Comparisons, 1995.

Pavan-Langston D. Manual of Ocular Diagnosis and Therapy (3rd ed). Boston: Little, Brown, 1991.

Pau H. Differential Diagnosis of Eye Diseases. Philadelphia: Saunders, 1978.

Roy FP. Ocular Differential Diagnosis (4th ed). Philadelphia: Lea & Febiger, 1989.

Roy FP. Ocular Syndromes and Systemic Diseases (2nd ed). Philadelphia: Saunders, 1989.

Rubin L. Optometrist's Desk Reference Book (3rd ed). Boston: Butterworth, 1988.

Sanford JP. Guide to Antimicrobial Therapy 1994. Dallas: Antimicrobial Therapy, 1994.

Schlaegel TF. Symptoms and Signs of Uveitis. In TD Duane (ed), Clinical Ophthalmology. Vol. 4. Philadelphia: Harper & Row, 1984.

Schlaegel TF. Etiologic Diagnosis of Uveitis. In TD Duane (ed), Clinical Ophthalmology. Vol. 4. Philadelphia: Harper & Row, 1984.

Speicher CE, Smith JW. Choosing Effective Laboratory Tests. Philadelphia: Saunders, 1983.

Steinsapir KD, Goldberg RA. Traumatic optic neuropathy. Surv Ophthalmol 1994;38:487–518.

Thompson S, Corbett JJ, Cox TA. How to measure the relative afferent pupillary defect. Surv Ophthalmol 1981;26:1.

Vaughan D, Asbury T, Tabbara KF. General Ophthalmology (13th ed). Norwalk, CT: Appleton & Lange, 1992.

von Noorden GK. Binocular Vision and Ocular Motility. St. Louis: Mosby, 1990.

Walsh JB, Gold A (ed). Physician's Desk Reference for Ophthalmology (22nd ed). Oradell, NJ: Medical Economics, 1994.

Walsh TJ. Neuro-ophthalmology: Clinical Signs and Symptoms (3rd ed). Philadelphia: Lea & Febiger, 1992.

Weinberg DV, Murphy R, Naughton K. Combined daily therapy with intravenous ganciclovir and foscarnet for patients with recurrent cytomegalovirus retinitis. Am J Ophthalmol 1994;117:776–782.

White P, Scott C. Contact Lenses and Solutions Summary. Supplement to Contact Lens Spectrum. December 1994.

Wilson LA, Sexton RS. Laboratory Aids in Diagnosis. In TD Duane (ed), Clinical Ophthalmology. Vol. 4. Philadelphia: Harper & Row, 1984.

Wilson LA. Bacterial Corneal Ulcers. In TD Duane (ed), Clinical Ophthalmology. Vol. 4. Philadelphia: Harper & Row, 1984.

Index